DIABETIC MANUAL

By ELLIOTT P. JOSLIN, M.D., Sc.D.

*The Late Clinical Professor of Medicine, Emeritus, Harvard
Medical School; Formerly, Medical Director, George F. Baker
Clinic at New England Deaconess Hospital; Consulting
Physician, Boston City Hospital; Honorary President, International Diabetes Federation; Honorary President, American Diabetes Association, President, Diabetes Foundation, Inc.*

Tenth Edition, Illustrated

for the Patient

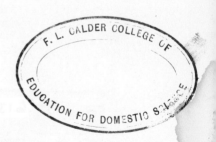

LEA & FEBIGER • PHILADELPHIA

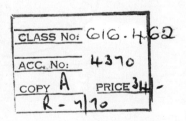
Library of Congress Card Catalog Number: 59-12083

Printed in the United States of America

34/-

37

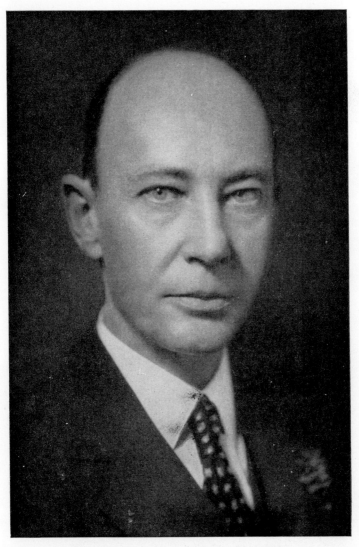

DR. GEORGE RICHARDS MINOT, 1885–1950

Saved by Insulin—Co-discoverer of the Treatment of
Pernicious Anemia.   Nobel Laureate 1934

Disce ut semper victurus
Vive ut cras moriturus.

Learn as if you were to live forever
Live as if you were to die tomorrow.

Isidore, Archbishop of Seville.
c. 570–636.

PREFACE

IT IS seldom a diabetic patient returns whom I have treated as well as I might, or one who has followed treatment as well as he could. Diabetes is a serious disease and deserves the best effort of doctor and patient from beginning to end. Sixty years of experience with diabetics convinces me that aggressive and continuous treatment with strict control of the disease pays.

To hasten better times for diabetics the creation of Hospital Teaching Clinics to which they can go at lessened hospital expense for control of the disease at present offers the greatest return for the money expended. Such clinics should be established all over the world. From these centers would radiate information on the detection and prevention of diabetes as well as advice for the care of the individual. Under no circumstances should the relatives of a diabetic become fat, thereby adding still more to the influence of heredity and to the chance of acquiring the disease.

Improvements in the treatment of diabetics are more likely to occur in the immediate future than ever before, because the tools for research are so much superior to those hitherto employed and there are so many more highly trained workers. Diabetics! Keep alive to profit by the new discoveries which you and your relatives and friends are fostering through liberal contributions for research.

Recognition of the importance of diabetes is increasing. At least three times as many diabetics are alive as formerly and many times as many are regarded as productive workers and are eligible for life insurance. Each diabetic who lives an honest diabetic day helps all other diabetics in the world to earn a living.

It would be a major contribution to the statistics of diabetes in this country if each patient would notify his or her doctor on New Year's Day that he or she was still alive.

I hope doctors and patients will find the enclosed identification and diet cards so useful they will be carried at all times, and one more wish—that all who read this book will take to heart the principles of Naunyn, that Nestor of Diabetes, (see pages 153–154), which I have tried to follow for sixty years.

To the doctors who have trusted me with their cases, to nurses, patients, my associates in the Joslin Clinic, to the Statistical Bureau of the Metropolitan Life Insurance Company, the United States Public Health Service and innumerable friends, and especially in the rewriting of this tenth edition to Miss Anna C. Holt, I am indebted, as well as to my cooperative publishers, the Messrs. Lea & Febiger, who have had the temerity to issue twenty editions of my two books.

ELLIOTT P. JOSLIN

BOSTON, MASS.

CONTENTS

Diabetic Manual

1

DIABETES

INTRODUCTION

If you are a diabetic, remember you are not the only one. There are about three million others in the United States alone and the majority of them lead useful lives. Their number is increasing, (1) because diabetics are living so much longer, (2) are having so many more children and (3) diabetes is chiefly a disease of older people and the average duration of life of the entire population is lengthening. Therefore, face the facts, accept the situation, study the disease and become master of your fate. By so doing you are sure to help those less fortunate and may defer or even prevent the onset of diabetes in other members of your own family.

Prevent Diabetes

Prevent it, but how? Diabetes is hereditary. Yes, but it takes two to make a diabetic. Therefore, a diabetic must not marry another diabetic and by all means should try to avoid marrying into a diabetic family. That is difficult, I will own, because one person in four inherits the tendency. Fortunately, there is another way to prevention, namely, don't be overweight. Above the age of thirty, 80 to 90 per cent of most diabetics are fat before they develop the disease. Consequently, if you are a relative of a diabetic, don't be fat because thereby you increase immeasurably your chances of getting diabetes. Indeed, to be stylish don't be fat under any circumstances and if you wish to be really up to date, plan not to have a big baby because the woman who has an infant weighing 12 or more pounds at birth stands a 100 per cent chance later of herself becoming a diabetic.

Diabetes is a disease in which part of the food escapes use by the body and is lost as sugar in the urine. If the patient stops overeating and eats less sugar and starch, most of the symptoms of diabetes will vanish. To make up for the loss of sugar and starch in the diet, one may need to take more meat, fish, eggs, cheese (protein) or a little more fat such as cream, butter, oil and fat meat. Should the urine not become sugar free with this moderate change of diet, it is wiser to take insulin. Pills of various kinds are useful in a few elderly people but unlike insulin, they are not a normal constituent of the body, they are foreign to it. If you take insulin you are replacing what the body lacks; if you take oral drugs, as far as present knowledge goes, you are lowering the blood sugar and possibly helping otherwise.

Insulin was discovered in 1921 by Banting and Best in Toronto, Canada. It came into use the next year, and from then on, it has altered the entire outlook for diabetics. It is one of the greatest discoveries in medicine. Protamine insulin was devised in 1936 by Hagedorn of Copenhagen. Two years later it was improved by Scott and Fisher of Toronto through the inclusion of zinc, and again improved by Hagedorn as NPH insulin, so that one dose replaces three or four doses of the original insulin. Globin insulin and Lente insulin are other varieties. In addition to diet and insulin, exercise is a powerful aid in treatment. Without exercise it is far more difficult to keep the urine sugar free and blood sugar normal and so control the diabetes.

Not only does insulin free the urine of sugar, but it makes possible the return of health to the patient and the prospect of a long life. Best states the "action of

insulin is to remove all signs and symptoms of diabetes . . ."[1]

The diet of a diabetic need not be severe or conspicuous. He should be able to eat without injury to
himself, either without or with the aid of insulin, at the
very least the equivalent of the food described below.
No one wants him to become fat.

BREAKFAST: Fruit, one portion; cereal and a slice of
bread and butter; 1 egg or, if he needs more nourishment, either 2 eggs or 1 egg with bacon.

LUNCH: Meat, fish or cheese; vegetables, unrestricted
in quantity save the very starchy ones such as potato
and corn; 1 slice of bread; fruit for dessert.

DINNER: A meal similar to that at noon but rather
more abundant and usually containing a salad.

During the day at least $\frac{3}{4}$ pint of milk and not over
one ounce of butter. Clear broths, coffee, tea, cocoa
shells and cracked cocoa can be taken without allowance
for food content.

Diabetes Widespread

Diabetes is a common disease in middle life, but unusual in the young and rare in children. Among 2500
children one finds but 1 diabetic, but above the age of
sixty-five years, 1 man in 70 will have it and 1 woman
in 45[2]. A hundred years ago Bouchardat[3] in France
wrote: "I do not believe I am wrong in saying that
among twenty men between the ages of forty to sixty
years, belonging to legislative assemblies, in noted

---

[1] Best: Research Defense Soc. Pub., 26, Nr. 3, 1938.
[2] These figures are based on a National Health Survey made in
1935–36.
[3] Bouchardat: De la Glycosurie ou Diabète Sucré, Paris, 1883,
p. 180.

learned societies, occupying high positions in commerce and finance, and even in the army, one is sure to find a glycosuric." It was found as a result of a diabetes survey in 1947, in Oxford, Massachusetts, that about 1 in 70 had diabetes. The Oxford study doubled our estimate of the number of diabetics in this country, but undoubtedly it will more than double the yearly efforts, financial and otherwise, expended in overcoming the disease. It is as frequent in Negroes and Indians as among the white population, and perhaps most frequent of all in the Jewish people, because of intermarriage and obesity. The percentage among Hebrews and the colored race is surely decreasing because the younger generations weigh less. In the next 10 years statistics from Israel will probably disclose much new information.

Today we hear more about diabetes in children than formerly, because they live so long. The Metropolitan Life Insurance Company tells me from a study of my cases that a diabetic child of ten years already has a life expectancy of forty-five years. The younger the diabetic at onset of diabetes, the longer the individual has to live. More than twice as many die above the age of sixty years with diabetes as under the age of twenty years. For one individual who develops diabetes under forty, there are two who acquire it above forty years. However, diabetes seldom occurs in persons over forty years of age unless they are fat. In young or old there must be an hereditary element, although one cannot always find it. The influence of heredity alone may not be strong enough to make the disease develop unless the individual helps to bring it on by overeating or the tolerance for carbohydrate is lowered during pregnancy, by infections or complicating disease of the thyroid, pituitary or adrenal glands.

Diabetes is universal and its incidence is highest where the average age is greatest, females predominate, diet is most easily obtained with resulting obesity, and medical supervision for its detection is the most thorough. Between 1951 and 1954, with notable economic improvement, the incidence of diabetes in Italy rose 30 per cent, but in the United States remained about constant. In Italy during 1954 the incidence was two-thirds that of the United States.

Death from diabetes, pure and simple, is needless, if the patient follows the rules of treatment. Most of the complications of diabetes are avoidable if patients will control it and take common-sense precautions. Not a single death from diabetes in a person under thirty years of age was reported in the city of Boston during 1957.

Object of Treatment

The object of the treatment of diabetes is to prevent its complications by avoiding an increase of sugar in the blood with the loss of sugar in the urine. This is accomplished: (1) by altering the diet so that the patient will take less than usual of sugar and starch, and in general by eating only moderate quantities of all foods; (2) by exercise which favors the burning up of sugar in the muscles; (3) by insulin which is a hormone (a chemical substance) made out of cells of the pancreas of any animal and, passing into the blood stream, excites other cells in the body to activity. This manufactured insulin replaces the insulin which the diabetic's pancreas has ceased to produce in sufficient quantity. Oral drugs lower the sugar in the blood. Treatment with diet alone was formerly unsatisfactory, because the diet was often too strict for comfort or occasionally for life. The patients were sometimes too weak even to benefit from exercise. The discovery of insulin was a great boon, because with its help the patient could eat all he needed to enable him to work or play and to become a normal member of society. Think of all that Dr. George R.

Minot, himself a diabetic, did for patients with pernicious anemia through his contribution to the discovery of how it could be helped. Perhaps he was my most noted patient. At all events, I always have felt that his intense study of his own diet gave him courage to feed raw liver to his patients.

Sugar is present in the urine (glycosuria) in untreated diabetes and there is also an excess in the blood (hyperglycemia). This is due to the body having lost the power to use the food which has been eaten. Most of the sugar which leaks through the kidneys into the urine comes from sugar and starch (carbohydrate), but some can be formed out of meat, fish, eggs and cheese (protein) and a little from pure fat. Healthy persons do not have sugar in the urine, because the secretion of insulin by the pancreas, (a gland in the abdomen often called the sweetbread), is a prime factor in the storage of sugar in the liver and muscles as animal starch (glycogen), and makes possible its change to body fat or its use for energy as fast as it is formed.

The Advantages of Diabetes Over Other Chronic Diseases

It is perfectly true that diabetes is a chronic disease, but, unlike rheumatism and cancer, it is painless when controlled, unlike tuberculosis, it is clean and not contagious, and in contrast to many diseases of the skin, it is not unsightly. Moreover, it is susceptible to treatment, and any downward course of a patient can be promptly checked. Effective treatment, however, rests in the hands of the patient. It is by diet and exercise as well as by insulin or oral drugs. Patients with the will to win and those who know the most, conditions being equal, can live the longest. There is no disease in which an understanding by the patient of the methods of treatment avails as much. Brains count. But knowledge alone will not save the diabetic. This is a disease which tests the character of the patient, and for success in withstanding it, in addition to wisdom, he must possess common sense, honesty, self-control and courage. These qualities are as essential along with insulin as without insulin. About three thousand of my patients have actually lived longer with diabetes than they were expected to live without it, and far longer than their fat friends, both diabetic and non-diabetic, whose obesity led to premature death by way of heart or kidneys. For the diabetic this is a demonstration and a challenge. To such patients we give an Expectation of Life Medal. See pages 206 and 210.

Diabetics, young and old, have had outstanding careers and have held high positions in war and peace. In June, 1948, one of my diabetic boys graduated as valedictorian in a large Eastern college and was also president of his class, and later like another patient, was a Rhodes scholar.

Definition of Diabetes Mellitus

Diabetes is a chronic hereditary disease in which there is an increase of sugar in the blood (hyperglycemia) and an excretion of sugar in the urine (glycosuria); it is dependent upon disease of the pancreas, particularly of groups of cells called the islands of Langerhans which have close connection with several other glands in the body; the secretion of the islands of Langerhans—insulin—not only promotes the normal storage of glycogen (animal starch) in the liver, muscles and skin and the combustion of glucose (sugar) in the tissues, but also exerts a control upon the transformations of protein and fat.

My rule in the treatment of diabetes is to consider any patient who has sugar in the urine demonstrable by any of the common tests to have diabetes mellitus and to treat him as a diabetic until the contrary is proved.

Occasionally an individual has sugar in the urine and yet the sugar in the blood is not above normal. Such a patient is not considered to have diabetes, but to have renal—kidney—glycosuria. Rarely a patient shows a positive test for sugar in the urine, which is due to other varieties of sugar—pentose, levulose or lactose. This is harmless. The quantity is always small and in such cases the blood sugar is normal.

The development of diabetes may be gradual or acute and with or without symptoms. It is fortunate that the disease can be so readily discovered, for unlike many diseases whose beginnings can be detected only by specialists or disclosed by the help of elaborate and expensive methods, such as the *x*-rays, diabetes can be easily and promptly recognized by any physician who will be on the watch for it and will examine the urine of his patient for sugar. Responsibility for early detection of the disease among relatives must be shared by the patient with the physician. In the treatment of a diabetic one always has the family in mind. The subsequent behavior of the disease and the effect of treatment are also easily regulated by simple urinary examinations and simple tests for the percentage of sugar in the blood; herein the diabetic has a great advantage over many patients with other diseases.

Symptoms

The symptoms of diabetes are thirst, hunger and the passage of an increased quantity of urine (polydipsia, polyphagia and polyuria) with loss of weight and strength. Itching of the skin, particularly about the genitals, is common. There is no one symptom always present and indeed there are many diabetics who notice no symptoms. This is the reason it is so desirable for everybody to have routine examinations of the urine at least once a year and always when indisposed, because it is only in this way that all cases will be discovered and found out so early that treatment can begin promptly. The eyesight may be affected and occasionally the nerves show trouble by pains or difficulty in moving certain muscles. But these are complications rather than a part of the disease. A properly treated case of diabetes should feel well and have no symptoms. The responsibility for maintaining this favorable state must rest in large measure upon the patient himself. He must learn the diet, the dose of insulin and the amount of exercise which are best for him and must constantly control his condition by the examination of his urine. He is his own nurse and chemist, but if he tries to be his own doctor, he will come to grief. To acquire the requisite knowledge requires diligent study, but the prize offered is worth while, for it is nothing less than life itself.

The diabetic problem for the doctor has not been simplified with the passing of the years. Nowadays, he must educate his patients to control their diabetes and thus protect themselves from those unnecessary complications which usually occur most often after a decade or two of the disease. Once we tried to keep the breath of life in our diabetics for five years, but now we try to maintain their vigor for over fifty years.

Source of Urinary Sugar

The sugar in the urine of diabetic patients is derived from their food, and chiefly from that consumed within the preceding twenty-four hours and also from the breakdown of body tissue. The effects of a meal begin to show within ten minutes after eating by an increase of sugar in the blood and the appearance of sugar in the urine. Most of the sugar in the urine comes from carbohydrates, but also can be derived from protein and fat. A fasting individual in reality is always eating

2

because, cannibal-like, he is consuming his own body. Thus even without taking food into his mouth a severe diabetic may form sugar and show it in the urine. In such a case the sugar is formed from protein and fat, because there is little carbohydrate stored as such in the body. It seldom amounts to as much as three-quarters of a pound and is nearly all exhausted within 24 hours if a diabetic goes without food.

Test of Successful Treatment

Improvement in diabetes takes place when the sugar in the blood is normal and the urine is free from sugar. The annoying symptoms of the untreated diabetic then vanish. Under such conditions the pancreas increases the utilization of the sugar and starch in the diet. Conversely, if the urine is not free from sugar, the patient is generally only holding his own, or more likely is growing worse. Professor Naunyn of Germany, who for a generation was perhaps the leading specialist in diabetes, wrote in his book: "Above all, it is important for the early cases that the diabetes right at its start be treated so energetically that if possible the control of the glycosuria be attained. From my experience I consider it very probable that among the early strictly treated patients who in the beginning appear as severe but later on run a favorable course there are many who are indebted to this early strict treatment; and, on the other hand, there cannot be the slightest doubt that the ultimately severely coursing cases in the great majority of instances are those who underwent energetic treatment not until late if ever."

The Blood Sugar and Its Value in Diagnosis and Treatment

Examination of the blood for sugar gives valuable information in the treatment of diabetes. The total quantity of pure sugar (not sugar and glycogen) actually in the *blood* of the entire body is surprisingly small. Before meals it amounts to about 1 teaspoonful (5 grams); and after meals, if the pancreas with its insulin did not prevent its rising above a scant 2 teaspoonfuls, sugar would leak through the kidneys into the urine and the individual would be a diabetic. The normal percentage of sugar in the blood is 0.10 per cent,

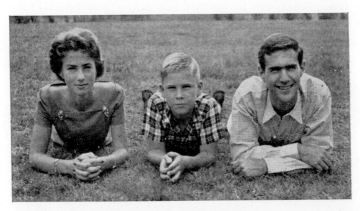

Fig. 1.—The mother of these children developed diabetes at the age of eight years in 1921 and literally through treatment by starvation was kept alive until insulin was available in 1922. She was married in 1935. After seventeen years of diabetes a son was born, two years later a daughter and in 1946 another son. The father is a non-diabetic from a non-diabetic family. In 1958 after 37 years of diabetes, she went on a trip to Paris, Brussels and London.

(usually stated as 100 mg.), but after a meal it may rise to about 0.15 per cent (150 mg.) without sugar appearing in the urine. The adjustment of the mechanism by which the insulin regulates the quantity of sugar in the blood within these narrow limits is truly wonderful. It does this through the effect of insulin, supplied by the pancreas or injected, which changes the soluble sugar into insoluble starch (glycogen) and stores it in the liver, muscles and other tissues, or else favors its combustion to give us energy.

Further simplification of a test for sugar in the blood, which will make it as available for doctor and patient as is the test for sugar in the urine, would mark a tremendous advance in treatment, and can be expected.

The sugar in the blood usually rises above normal before sugar appears in the urine. Consequently if information can be learned about the blood sugar, one often anticipates the information which an examination of the urine alone would show. The knowledge about the blood sugar is still fragmentary, and it must be acknowledged that many cases of diabetes have lived comfortably without a single blood sugar estimation. However, analyses of the blood sugar are of great value, and without them errors in diagnosis and treatment sometimes occur. Of the 4,219 children treated by our group, I have known several to take insulin for more than a year when they did not need it, and with one of these I made the mistake. Although it did her no harm, I am always glad to receive Helen's New Year's card. It is the patient who did not receive insulin who suffers.

2

CONTROL OF DIABETES
AND
WHY I BELIEVE IT WORTH WHILE

MY MOTHER's diabetes was recognized in 1900. She was my Case No. 8. Naturally, I went to Strassburg to learn from Naunyn, the Nestor of diabetes, how to treat her. Following his methods and with a relatively low-carbohydrate, high-fat diet, which I can truthfully say I never knew her to break, the 6 per cent sugar soon disappeared and she lived healthfully and cheerfully for 13 years with her diabetes which was as long as she was expected to live without it. It is true, complications developed—a carbuncle, pneumonia, intermittent claudication and finally a cerebro-vascular accident with a lethal (kind) pneumonia. This case was the first to teach me that control of the disease paid. Think of the effect of that one life upon the 52,000 which have come under my observation during 60 years of practice. Emerson's lines which she loved are certainly appropriate—

> "Little thinks, in the field, yon red-cloaked clown
> Of thee from the hill-top looking down;
> The heifer that lows in the upland farm,
> Far-heard, lows not thine ear to charm;
> The sexton, tolling his bell at noon,
> Deems not that great Napoleon
> Stops his horse, and lists with delight,
> Whilst his files sweep round yon Alpine height;
> Nor knowest thou what argument
> Thy life to thy neighbor's creed has lent."

From Emerson: "Each and All."

(21)

In the Naunyn Era, 1897-1914, diabetic coma was responsible for 64 per cent of my patients who died. It was toward the end of that era when Dr. F. M. Allen, to whom I shall feel eternally grateful, emphasized the value of undernutrition in treatment and soon after Petrén in Sweden and we here noted that if our patients entered a hospital without coma they did not acquire it while in the hospital. Previously as a House Officer at the Massachusetts General Hospital in 1894-96, I noted the opposite was frequently the case. Control of diabetes was worthwhile. The slogan was to make diabetes as safe in the home as in the hospital. In fact, the percentage of deaths from coma fell in the next eight years to 42 per cent.

Then came insulin and the prospect was so overpowering that when I think of those days I am reminded of Keats' lines. See p. 27. It may be sentimental to quote so much poetry but anyone who has watched every diabetic child he had treated die and has lived through the period of coma and gangrene and later inanition so extreme that it cannot better be described than in the words of the prophet Ezekiel, See p. 37, would pardon an expression of sentiment because without it how could one have struggled ahead.

As yet we have not begun to fathom what insulin can do in diabetes if it is used to control it at its earliest appearance. But I do know from my own cases that coma has fallen from 64 per cent to 1 per cent; gangrene from 8 to 1 per cent and thanks to improvement in the care of infections, tuberculosis which once claimed fully 50 per cent of the deaths in large municipal hospitals, now has dropped almost to the vanishing point of 0.2 per cent in our own series. The control of diabetes which insulin made possible is obvious.

Again, the effects of control are shown because the average duration of life of our patients, which up to 1914, was 4.9 years now is 18 years. Children with onset in the first decade of life at first lived 1.2 years; now our recent fatal cases have survived 26 years. Eighty per cent of our patients with onset in childhood are alive. See Table 12, p. 208 and p. 252.

It would be unfair to claim that these reductions in mortality and the lengthening lives of patients were due wholly to control of the disease. Better sanitation, cleanliness, antibiotics, modern surgery have contributed much.

Other methods are available which show the effect of control, and one of these is illustrated by Amelia Peabody in her Life Expectancy Medal. See page 210. I suppose that upwards of 3000 of our patients have earned one by living longer with diabetes than they were expected to live without it. Scanning the histories of these individuals it is evident that unusual attention was paid to the diabetes, not only by the patients but by their doctors. Intelligence counted for much. By no means were the patients always in the upper classes of society. Many an individual in a modest home has earned our Medal.

The most striking argument for meticulous control and the one which led to the foundation of the Hospital Teaching Clinic is that of Sam R., Case 2419. He developed diabetes at the age of 14. For the next 7 years he had one of our diabetic nurses and obeyed her implicitly. The first years he lived on undernutrition diets which were followed to the letter. Gradually the dietetic tension eased. Everything that money could buy was at his disposal and that of his nurse. They flew their own airplane alone weekends from New Jersey to Cape Cod. They travelled to Europe and found 5 units of insulin could be dropped from the diet when tennis was played in the Bois de Boulogne. Eventually, he married and his prospective bride studied and practiced the details of treatment during 6 months before the wedding. When 25 years had elapsed since the onset of his diabetes, we discovered the patient was physically perfect—eyes, arteries, blood vessels, kidneys —and this led to the inauguration of the Quarter Century Victory Medal. See p. 211. Today he is 53 years old and a healthy, vigorous business man with

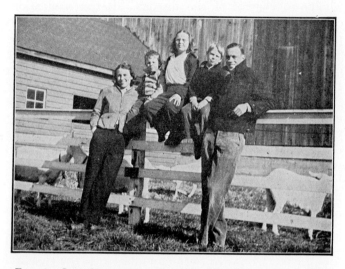

FIG. 2—Case No. 2419. The father of these three children developed diabetes at 14 years of age in 1920 and is an example of a thirty-nine-year duration diabetic child who had no signs or symptoms of arteriosclerosis, as certified in 1948 by *x*-ray and eye specialists and internists. His adherence to treatment has been exemplary. He is the first patient to receive Victory Medal. Note the two varieties of "kids."

3 children and a grandchild. His nurse and he and his family set the pace for our Victory Medal cases.

So far we have been able to award a Quarter Century Victory Medal to 85 individuals. As yet only those have been able to pass our criteria for a Medal whose diabetes is well controlled. A study of the histories of these medalists shows that from the beginning of the diabetes and particularly in its early years, their diabetes was carefully treated and at no time carelessly considered. The fact that no patient has yet been able to pass our criteria for a Victory Medal who did neglect his diabetes in the early days and later, is confirmation of the trust-worthiness of control.

Evidence of the value of control occurs in odd groups. In an English sanitarium for tuberculosis there were included 84 patients who were diabetics. Of these, only one patient died in a year and that one not of diabetes. In that sanitarium the diabetes as well as the tuberculosis was under control.

Bouchardat in 1883 says that he could not remember having ever seen a pregnant diabetic woman. In the early years of the century I know that pregnancy was rare and miscarriages were common. In all, two thousand pregnant diabetic women have come under our care, at least 1700 of them closely supervised by Dr. Priscilla White. Today the death of a pregnant diabetic woman is almost unknown. Here again. meticulous control saves the diabetic.[1]

The most distressing complication which our diabetics have at the present time occurs in the eyes. It is known as "retinitis proliferans." My colleague, Dr. Howard F. Root, has assembled 867 cases with this complication. He has studied these in great detail and recently reported upon them. In his analysis of these 867 cases, he has not found one in which the control of the diabetes was even good.

Do you wonder I believe that the control of diabetes is worth while? In this concept am I not aligning myself with those clinicians in the past whom we honor most because of their contribution to the treatment of dia-

[1]Dunlop of Edinburgh and Engleson in Sweden note similar findings in their recent publications.

betes—to Bouchardat, Naunyn, Cantani, Marañon, Umber, Grafe, Allen.

Insulin is a gift from Banting and Best aided by a mulitude of workers in countless laboratories searching endlessly to improve the effectiveness of this lifegiving substance.

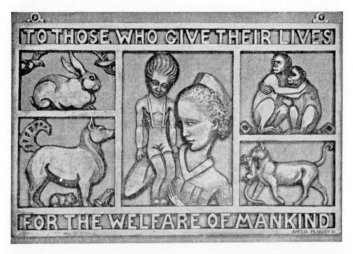

We doctors enjoy our medical practice, and our diabetic patients their lives, because of the victories over disease won by men and animals. There would be sorrow in our hearts if we were compelled to face a diabetic child without knowledge acquired by the scientific labors of physicians in many lands. But our minds linger as well on the animals who gave up their lives, not for their masters whom they loved but for diabetics whom they did not even know. And in recognition of what these lowly creatures have done we welcome the opportunity to insert a reproduction of the plaque created for us by Amelia Peabody and dedicated appropriately.

"TO THOSE WHO GIVE THEIR LIVES FOR THE WELFARE
OF MANKIND"

FIGURE 3

Keats' lines expressed my feelings when I learned of the discovery of insulin. I remained awake all night.

> "—Then felt I like some watcher of the skies
> When a new planet swims into his ken;
> Or like stout Cortez, when with eagle eyes
> He stared at the Pacific—and all his men
> Look'd at each other with a wild surmise—
> Silent, upon a peak in Darien."*

*A good many people, including my Central and South American friends, have been disturbed at the naming of Cortez by Keats in these memorable lines. Through the courtesy of Mr. Milton E. Lord, Director of the Boston Public Library, I learn that as authoritative a presentation as there has been on Keats was that done by Amy Lowell. On page 181 of Volume I of her two volumes on *John Keats* there appears the following: ". . . Keats confused Balboa with Cortez, as Tennyson pointed out to Palgrave, but Keats's friends do not seem to have noticed the mistake. Hunt, in *Imagination and Fancy*, refers to Titian's portrait of Cortez, and says 'his "eagle-eyes" are from life, as may be seen by Titian's portrait of him.' Keats may have known the portrait, or not, but at any rate he put Cortez, probably by accident. It is no matter."

3

DIABETES, INSULIN AND ORAL DRUGS

IT IS not necessary to read this chapter to learn how to control one's diabetes. It is written to show how our knowledge of the disease has advanced and that it has been through careful, clinical and experimental investigations in many lands—Germany, England, France, Belgium, Italy, Russia, Canada, Denmark, the Argentine, Chile, and the United States, and in many other countries.

In India and Rome there are hints of a knowledge of diabetes, but Paracelsus, born two years before Columbus discovered America in 1492, was the first to record that if a measure of urine of a diabetic patient was evaporated to a syrupy consistency it yielded 4 ounces of solids which he thought to be salt. Due to his mistake the world waited about 150 years until Thomas Willis[1] (1621-1675) tasted the urine of a diabetic and found it wonderfully sweet as if "imbued with honey." In 1775 Matthew Dobson, (England) proved by fermenting the urine that the sweet taste was actually due to sugar. John Rollo, also of England, in 1796, only four years before my grandfather was born, was the first to treat diabetics by diet and gave them animal food and vegetables such as our 3 and 6 per cent carbohydrate vegetables. In France, Bouchardat, the most celebrated diabetes clinician in the world (1806-1886) associated

[1]Thomas Willis was educated and taught for a time in Oxford, England. In Oxford, Massachusetts, the first intensive study of the frequency of diabetes based on examinations of urine and blood of the inhabitants was made. Here also is the Clara Barton Birthplace Camp for diabetic girls which originated in 1932.

the pancreas with diabetes, and Minkowski[1] and von Mering in Germany in 1889 proved diabetes was concerned with this gland, because when they removed it from a dog, severe diabetes occurred. In 1921 Banting and Best found that an extract of special cells in the pancreas, when injected into a diabetic, would control the disease. These cells were first described in 1869 by Langerhans in Germany and named after him, islands of Langerhans, but their significance as being responsible for diabetes was first noted by Opie in Baltimore and Ssobolew in Russia. The work of Banting and Best, who made an extract of these cells (1921), was done in the laboratory of Professor J. J. R. Macleod of Toronto, Canada. Later, with the help of Professor J. B. Collip, a biochemist, the active principle of the extract was refined and named insulin. On account of the discovery of insulin the Nobel Prize in Medicine was bestowed upon Banting and Macleod.

F. G. Banting was a young orthopedic surgeon with zeal for research undampened by four years of service at the front. He received the assistance of his friend, C. H. Best, who was trained in physiological research and who later entered the medical school. Dr. Charles H. Best is now Professor of Physiology at the University of Toronto, but by helping Banting discover insulin he proved that a medical student was *ipso facto* an investigator and deserved to be regarded as such.

Realizing that the action of insulin, although wonderful, lasted only a few hours and was also unlike nature in that it caused sudden and often serious falls, of the sugar in the blood, Hagedorn in Copenhagen, Denmark, sought to remedy these defects. For this purpose he utilized protamine, discovered in 1868 by Miescher, in Germany, in fish sperm and in the nuclei of cells and studied by Kossel in the last years of the nineteenth century. Experimenting with many protamines, he

[1] Born in Axolotl, a small town near Kovno (Kaunas) in Russia.

found one which would cause a precipitation of insulin. By adjusting the reaction of this solution with an alkali to that of the body, the resulting compound was absorbed so slowly that it acted twice as long as insulin alone. Still later Scott and Fisher, in Canada, observed that they could prolong the action for more than

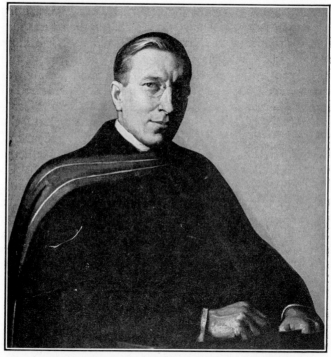

Fig. 4.—Sir Frederick G. Banting, M.D., K.C.B.E.

a day by the addition of an almost infinitesimal quantity of zinc. By these measures and by the invention of a modification of protamine zinc insulin (NPH insulin) by Hagedorn, the necessity for injections of insulin in the treatment of diabetes was reduced to once in twenty-four hours.

The next notable advance in the diabetic story relates to investigations upon the pituitary gland—the so-called master gland—in the center of the brain. Stimulated by earlier experiments of Houssay in the Argen-

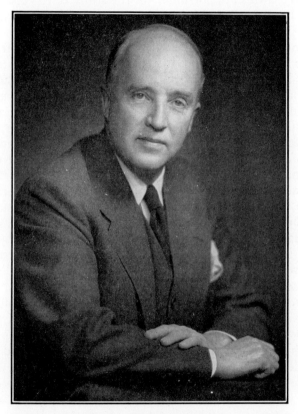

Fig. 5.—Charles H. Best.

tine and Evans in California and others to a lesser degree, Young in England produced diabetes in dogs by repeated injections of an extract of the anterior pituitary gland. Eventually it was found that the injections had destroyed the islands of Langerhans in the pancreas. Since the rest of the gland was uninjured it was possible now to study diabetes in an animal without the removal of so essential a gland, and this represented a fresh opportunity for the study of the disease.

The next, and third, achievement was in 1936 when Dunn, Sheehan and McLetchie in Glasgow, Scotland, found that a drug, alloxan (which can be derived from uric acid), when injected into a rabbit would destroy the beta cells which make the insulin in the islands of Langerhans in the pancreas. Almost simultaneously Goldner and Gomori in Chicago and Cabell Bailey and Orville Bailey in Boston proved that such animals became diabetic. This raised the problem: if a chemical can cause diabetes, does such a chemical exist in the human body, how can one detect it, and how neutralize its action? We have now experimental animals—rabbits, rats, dogs, cats, monkeys, pigeons, turtles—made diabetic by alloxan with which we can study the disease. So far alloxan has not been found in the human body but its precursor, uric acid, has been although it was shown by Griffiths in Australia that uric acid would not cause diabetes unless glutathione was reduced in the diet. Think of it! Alloxan is a selective drug. When introduced into an animal it attacks 1/14,000 part of the body and produces diabetes. How wonderful it would be if it was the cause of the disease in humans and we could thus determine those of a diabetic's relatives who were thus susceptible to the disease and how to destroy it. Certainly Griffiths in Australia has brought nearer this possibility by his discovery of uric acid diabetes as a result of a deficient quantity of glutathione.

> "If you can look into the seeds of time,
>   And say which grains will grow and which will not."

The year 1940 saw another trail of progress opened into the unexplored diabetic regions. Haist, Campbell and Best in Toronto learned that they could prevent a dog developing diabetes by injections of anterior pituitary extract if they treated him at the same time with insulin or if they fasted him beforehand or kept him on a fat diet. Moreover, Lukens and Dohan in Philadelphia found that they could cure a cat, similarly made diabetic for several months, by keeping the blood sugar normal with the use of insulin. Of course these experiments are confined to animals, but they are almost breath-taking in significance, because they raise the question of a cure of diabetes.

The fourth method of producing diabetes is, so far as the patient is concerned, perhaps the most suggestive of all. Dohan and Lukens at the Cox Metabolic Research Institute in Philadelphia artificially kept the blood sugar of a cat high for two weeks, whereupon they found diabetes appeared. As in all other experimental types of diabetes the islands of Langerhans were injured. The moral is plain. If a healthy cat with a sound pancreas will become diabetic, when exposed to a high blood sugar, how carefully should a diabetic with an unsound pancreas avoid it.

Diabetics! Take this lession to heart! Keep your urine sugar-free, your blood sugar normal and your diabetes controlled and thus protect your pancreas and thereby keep alive to profit by some new discovery.

The Pancreas and Its Islands of Langerhans

Diabetes is due to something wrong with the pancreas. This gland has a double action. It forms a digestive juice which, as a matter of fact, is the most important digestive juice in the body and this it discharges into the bowel just beyond the stomach; and, second, it produces insulin which is discharged into the blood, and this regulates the use of the sugar formed from the food. In animals the pancreas is known as the

3

sweetbread and lies behind the stomach near the liver. The pancreatic digestive juice is manufactured throughout the gland, but insulin is formed by collections of cells which occur in groups named the islands of Langerhans after the young doctor in Berlin who described them in 1869. It is possible experimentally to produce diabetes by removing more than nine-tenths of the pancreas, because then the few islands remaining are overworked, degenerate and cease to make the insulin which regulates the action of the sugar and starch. In man for some reason as yet unknown, the islands of Langerhans may become diseased or cease to function and diabetes appears. If the diabetic patient could secure a new pancreatic gland, would he be cured? Perhaps, but I think this is not certain because other glands may also be involved. Fortunately, among my 52,000 patients showing sugar in the urine I have never found one who was a 100 per cent diabetic. There has always been something left to build upon.

With this in mind, in 1944, Brush found by a study of children soon after the onset of their diabetes that if he overtreated them with insulin, thus resting their own pancreas by making unnecessary the production of insulin, as Umber had done with older patients, he could bring about a remission of the disease so that some of these children remained sugar free with a few or no units of insulin. Cures were not permanent, but hope was raised and still exists with every fresh case of diabetes in young and old that by intensive overtreatment with insulin some of the uninjured cells of the pancreas will be spared and so the disease kept in a still milder stage. More and more such attempts in young and old are being reported. Might it not be that the cases not quite diabetic—unclassified glycosurics—by being warned against eating excess carbohydrate and against obesity, were helped and as a result remained for years without showing frank diabetes? These borderline cases were once the bane of the doctor, the worry of life insurance examiners and a nuisance to themselves because they did not know whether they really were diabetic. Now these cases, of whom 2000 were studied by Dr. Marble, have shown that after 20 years only about 10 per cent became diabetic. "The stone which the builders rejected has become the head of the corner." Today, all borderline cases should be treated rigorously. Dr. Marble's cases who became diabetic were chiefly those who had a diabetic heredity, were overweight or of Jewish origin.

Insulin is prepared from the islands of Langerhans of the pancreas of various animals. Protamine insulin is insulin to which protamine is joined. At present protamine insulin is dispensed with the addition of zinc and is designated sometimes by its full name—protamine zinc insulin (PZI). Globin, Lente and NPH insulins are intermediate in action between PZI and regular (RI) and crystalline insulin (CI).

Insulin is prepared for general use dissolved in a liquid. The dose is measured in units. One unit of insulin when injected into a diabetic will enable him to utilize 1 or considerably more grams additional carbohydrate. Apparently the power of insulin varies in different patients and under different conditions with the same patient. Therefore, one must always proceed cautiously when administering the first dose. The number of units given in a day to a patient usually is between 10 and 50 units and if a clear solution (regular or crystalline) is employed, it is divided between one, two, three or four injections. Protamine zinc insulin is given in about the same quantity but only once a day because of its prolonged effect. In about half the cases both the quick- and slow-acting insulins are given at the same time before breakfast. The normal pancreas produces daily about 50 units.

If an excess of insulin is given, the blood sugar falls

below the normal of 0.10 (100 mg.) per cent and symptoms appear which are known as an "insulin reaction." The most striking of these are hunger, sweating and trembling and, unless treatment is instituted, unconsciousness may result. Nausea and headache are not uncommon symptoms with an excess of protamine insulin. Fortunately these symptoms quickly subside and disappear if the patient is given a little carbohydrate, such as the juice of an orange, a few teaspoonfuls of corn syrup or an equal quantity of sugar. Two lumps of sugar should always be carried by the patient.

Symptoms similar to those following an overdose of insulin occur with normal individuals after extreme exertion or when deprived of food. Along with those mentioned are nervousness, weakness, faintness, double vision, and dizziness. Occasionally the person is irritable, hilarious or irrational. Before the importance of a low blood sugar was known, athletes often had such symptoms. More often than we realize, a healthy person four or five hours after meals has a low blood sugar percentage, and in consequence behaves as does a diabetic during an insulin reaction. When any individual is hungry and out of sorts before a meal, I often wonder if his blood sugar is low. No one ever tries to sell anything or to raise money before a meal. Even if the prospective victim must pay for his dinner, the chances are better for making a sale or obtaining a subscription after a meal. My classmate, Harvey Cushing, used to say one should remember in raising money that the stomach is nearer the heart than the head, but I will add that the maintenance of a normal quantity of sugar in the blood is even more important.

Insulin is a remedy which a patient can learn to administer to himself, but it is nevertheless true that it is primarily a remedy for the wise and not the foolish, be they patients or doctors. Everyone knows it requires brains to live long with diabetes, but to use insulin successfully requires more brains.

Insulin is a comfort to doctor and patient. Insulin has revolutionized diabetic treatment in more ways than one. It has given the diabetic more food, strength and weight, but it has also carried to the doctor and the patient a knowledge and respect for the diabetic diet and for exercise, such as has never before existed. If the diabetic wishes to get his money's worth for the insulin he injects, he realizes that he must know what and how much to eat.

Good health, not tolerable health, is the right of the diabetic today and this is the real justification for the use of insulin. When I think of what the diabetics were when I treated them in the days of undernutrition (1914-1922) and what they are now with insulin, I am reminded of the words of the Prophet Ezekiel about 2500 years ago. No truer description of the transformation which has taken place in the life of a diabetic patient can be found than in the account of his vision of the valley of dry bones. (Ezekiel xxxvii, 1–10.)

Oral Substitutes For Insulin

Ever since the discovery of insulin there has been the hope that a way could be found to give it by mouth instead of under the skin. So far, no such method has been discovered, but the new oral drugs which lower the blood sugar—hypoglycemic agents—are encouraging harbingers.

The story of the sulfonylureas, which contain no insulin, began in Montpellier, France in 1942. Here Jambon and Loubatières noticed that the symptoms shown by a typhoid fever patient when treated with a certain sulfonylurea, of bactericidal power, resembled those of a patient in an insulin reaction.

Clinical application of this substance did not begin

until 1954–1955, when Franke and Fuchs, experimenting with similar material in Germany, confirmed the blood-sugar-lowering power. Then Franke used it in the treatment of diabetes. Bertram in Hamburg carried out tests with it clinically on a large scale and proved that it lowered the blood sugar in certain diabetics, mostly those above the age of 40 years with relatively short duration of the disease. Presumably, these individuals had some remaining capacity for the production of insulin in their own pancreas, because they were taking less than 20 units, (surely less than 40 units) of insulin daily. The drug employed was named carbutamide (BZ55). In a small percentage of the cases using the drug there were unfavorable features such as skin rashes, allergic responses and a few instances of jaundice, with the possibility of other harmful effects on the liver.

A second and similar drug remains in the body for periods up to 10 to 12 hours and was called tolbutamide (Orinase). In 1957 it was released for use by prescription in the United States.

One of the chief advantages of these drugs is that the blood-sugar-lowering effect is gradual, does not go to extremes and severe insulin-like reactions are generally avoided.

Essential for their success is close adherance to the diet. The new drugs provide no license for dietary excesses.

These drugs should not be employed in surgery, pregnancy, in the presence of infections, in acidosis or in other serious complications. They should not be used in the juvenile type of diabetes. Unlike insulin, they are compounds *foreign* to the human body.

As to the prolonged effect of their use, as yet no one knows. So far, no proof exists that they lessen the appearance of diabetic complications in the eyes, blood vessels or kidneys. They are not habit forming and as far as is known do not lose their power of action in the course of time, and if they seem to do so, it may simply represent carelessness in following the diet.

The mode of action of Orinase and all others of the same (sulfonylurea) group is still unanswered. They do not act by way of the thyroid, pituitary or adrenal glands. Some research suggests that they probably do stimulate the production of insulin in any remaining islands of Langerhans capable of producing it, or possibly increase insulin potency. Others think that these drugs act on the liver. They may prevent the release of sugar. They do not store up carbohydrate in the muscles (glycogen) as does insulin.

Aside from carbutamide (BZ55) and tolbutamide (Orinase), there is another sulfonylurea drug, Diabinese (Chlorpropamide). This is about three times stronger in action than tolbutamide and more slowly excreted, thus remaining longer in the body so that it may accumulate in the course of days. This fact must be borne in mind and care taken in prescribing its use.

An even newer drug from the sulfonylurea family is now under investigation. This is called Metahexamide. It is said to be effective in very small doses and is thought to remain in the body for a period somewhat shorter than Diabinese.

All four of these drugs (BZ55, Orinase, Diabinese and Metahexamide) seem to work in the same type of patient, namely the newer and milder cases.

A different type of drugs called biguanides is now being investigated in many centers. These drugs are unlike the sulfonylureas both in chemical structure and chemical action. There is a series of these drugs called DBI, DBB, DBV. All are closely related to phenethyl-formamidinyliminourea, best known as DBI or Phenformin. These are strange drugs because, unlike the sulfonylureas, they are not effective in normal people. Clinical experience suggests that either they (1) increase the effectiveness of insulin (already present in the body or given by needle), or (2) in some way prevent an unknown substance from interfering with the normal action of insulin.

In the 1920's a guanidine drug called Synthalin was shown to lower the blood sugar levels. The use was abandoned because of reported toxic effects and because insulin was discovered. In large doses DBI appears to act in some ways like Synthalin because over-doses of both drugs cause some loss of appetite, nausea and vomiting.

Dr. Leo Krall of our group has been investigating many of these drugs and tells me that:

(1) The biguanide drugs lower blood sugar in a wide variety of patients, some whose diabetes was too severe to be helped by the other oral drugs.

(2) There is a high incidence of side effects but these are readily reversed by lowering the dose or omitting the drug.

(3) There has been no toxicity to date.

(4) The chief clinical usefulness of these drugs may be as a stabilizing agent in some of the severe and juvenile-onset diabetics who are difficult to regulate with insulin because of severe reactions.

We have tried carbutamide (BZ55) with more than 350 cases; tolbutamide (Orinase) with far more than 1500 cases; Diabinese with more than 125 cases; and DBI with over 300 cases. About 1 in 10 or 15 of our patients now under observation is being treated with one or the other of these preparations. I use Orinase in many cases, but not the other drugs. I think they should be employed by others in our group who are making a special study of these compounds. Writing as of May 1959, I do not believe it advisable for a patient doing well with insulin for 20 years or more to attempt to replace it with oral medication. "Don't swap horses in mid-stream."

Tolbutamide (Orinase) comes in half-gram doses. Gradually one can increase from 1 pill to 4 or 6 daily, at the same time proportionately reducing the insulin if this has been taken. Under close observation one can begin with 2 pills three times daily. The appearance of acetone, diacetic acid—acid-poisoning or ketosis—is a signal to stop their use, as is also the non-disappearance of sugar from the urine. *Under no circumstances* should testing of the urine during such an experimental period be dropped and it is dangerous to use these drugs except under the close supervision of a physician. Any severe illness or infection is a signal for immediate return to insulin. This is also true of an elevated blood sugar or increased glycosuria from any cause.

The discovery of these chemicals has resulted in an added respect for diet, exercise and reduction of excess weight in the treatment of diabetes. It has stimulated research to an enormous degree in order to explain how these drugs act and, incidentally, it has helped to explain some of the mechanisms of diabetes.

Certainly, all will agree that these drugs are harbingers of better days for diabetics, because many things heretofore taken for granted are being re-investigated. Newer drugs and methods of treatment are sure to be found. This new Experimental Era will lead not only to greater emphasis on diabetes but also will result in improved treatment.

4

QUESTIONS AND ANSWERS
FOR DIABETIC PATIENTS

In an "Author's Apology" for a well-known classic occurred certain lines which have influenced me in the preparation of this diminutive chapter. I only wish that my language was as simple and that it would say to my patients as has his to readers for nearly three hundred years—

> "Art thou forgetful? Wouldest thou remember
> From New-year's-day to the last of December?
> Then read my Fancies, they will stick like Burrs,
> And may be to the Helpless, Comforters."

THE DIABETIC should take no chances; along with a clean body and trained muscles he should have a mind prepared and alert, and temperament under control, because he depends upon his brains to make up in part for the loss of his pancreas. Diabetes lasts for life. Therefore, treatment should be arranged and carried out in such a way as to interfere as little as possible in the daily life. The patient must be taught the nature of his disease; how to combat it; how to avoid its complications. The sooner these three facts are learned the better.

1. QUESTION. What part of the body is at fault in diabetes?
ANSWER. The pancreas. Take it out and diabetes appears.

2. Q. What are the common symptoms?
A. Hunger, thirst and frequent urination, loss of weight and strength, and itching, local or general.

3. Q. How is the disease controlled?

A. By diet, exercise and insulin and in mild and uncomplicated cases, hopefully, by oral drugs.

4. Q. How is the urine tested for sugar?

A. Put 4 drops of urine in a test-tube and add a half teaspoonful Benedict's solution. Shake well and place in boiling water for five minutes. Colors after boiling: blue means no sugar; green shows a small amount; yellow a moderate amount; and orange or red a large amount of sugar. Several other simpler and more convenient tests are available such as Clinitest, Clinistix, Tes-Tape.

5. Q. How often should the urine be tested?

A. Always on rising; often upon retiring; occasionally before noon and night meals; and at any time, if in doubt about condition; or during any illness.

6. Q. Why is insulin given to a diabetic?

A. To replace the insulin which the pancreas has failed to produce and thus save food for body weight and body strength.

7. Q. Why do untreated diabetics grow thin?

A. They do not get enough value out of the food they eat to make up for that lost as sugar in the urine. (See pages 200–202, Fig. 25, p. 202.)

8. Q. Why are untreated diabetics thirsty?

A. They must drink sufficient liquids to dissolve the sugar which is escaping from the blood through the kidneys into the urine.

9. Q. How much sugar is lost in diabetes?

A. From a mere trace to 2 pounds in 24 hours.

10. Q.   How can a diabetic gain weight and strength?

A.   By preventing loss of sugar in the urine so as to get the benefit of what he eats. This is accomplished (1) through diet by limiting the quantity and quality of the food, (2) by the use of insulin or oral drugs, (3) by exercise which helps the body to utilize those foods which turn to sugar.

11. Q.   What foods are most likely to cause sugar in the urine?

A.   Carbohydrate foods. Those which contain sugar and starch. Cane sugar is the commonest sugar. A pure form of starch is corn starch. Fruits are almost entirely water and sugar, and vegetables are largely water and starch. Bananas, when green, contain nearly 20 per cent starch, but when ripened this changes to sugar. Starchy foods during digestion in the body rapidly change to sugar, and consequently sugar and starch are nearly interchangeable. Potatoes are 20 per cent starch, bread 50 to 60 per cent, and the flour out of which bread is made, being drier than the bread, contains about 70 per cent. Oatmeal is two-thirds starch, but other cereals contain more. Milk contains 5 per cent sugar. A small percentage of animal starch (glycogen) exists in liver. For carbohydrate in various foods see Tables 3, 4, 5, p. 65, 66, 67, Table 26, p. 287.

12. Q.   What other type of food may change to sugar in the body and appear as such in the urine?

A.   Protein. At least 58 per cent may undergo this change. Protein is the food from which muscles and tissues are made. It is therefore essential, and every person and every animal likes it. The cat will catch a mouse, because there is more protein in meat than in milk; the pony, Jouett, gladly comes for his bridle, and the timid sheep love to feed out of Carolyn's hand just because there is more protein in oats than in grass.

Examples of protein are lean of meat or fish, curd of milk, and white of egg. The yolk contains just as much protein as the white, but it is mixed with fat. Protein is also found in nuts and grains, and there is considerable in beans and peas, but very little in other vegetables, even potatoes, and almost none in fruits.

13. Q. What kind of food is least apt to change to sugar?

A. Fat. Theoreticaly only 10 per cent. Examples of fat in pure form are olive oil and lard. Butter and substitutes for it contain 85 per cent fat. Rich cream contains about 40 per cent fat, whereas milk may contain but 3 per cent. Common cheese is one-third fat. The percentage of fat in meat varies from that in fat bacon, in which the percentage occasionally rises to 80 per cent, to chicken, in which the percentage of fat is 3 per cent or less. In codfish and haddock the amount of fat is negligible, but in salmon it reaches 13 per cent. Nuts are rich in fat. Fat and carbohydrate are to a large extent interchangeable in the diet of the normal person. In northern climates fat forms a large part of the diet, while in the tropics it is replaced by carbohydrate. Today it is considered wiser to replace a part of the saturated butter fat and animal fat with an unsaturated vegetable fat, such as corn oil "Mazola", or saffron oil—see Table 26, p. 287.

14. Q. If fat hardly changes at all to sugar in the body, why does a diabetic not live upon fat alone?

A. (a) He would tire of it. (b) Fat does not contain protein and so would not replace the tissues of the body. (c) If fat replaces carbohydrates and protein in the diet to an extreme degree in a diabetic, acid poisoning (acidosis) develops and unless treated this leads to diabetic coma and death. Even normal dogs fed upon a diet consisting only of fat bacon die in a few months.

15. Q. What is the proof a diabetic is not controlling his disease and utilizing the food he eats?
A. Sugar in the urine, and increased sugar in the blood.

16. Q. What are the sources of sugar in the urine?
A. (1) Carbohydrate in the diet; (2) protein; (3) fat. A hundred grams of carbohydrate yield 100 grams of sugar; 100 grams of protein, 58 or more grams of sugar and 100 grams of fat 10 grams of sugar. In diabetes sugar may appear in the urine irrespective of the diet because it is derived from protein and fat of which the body is so largely composed. The body of the normal individual is made up of water, 58 per cent; protein, 16 per cent; fat, 21 per cent; carbohydrate, 1 per cent; minerals, 4 per cent. Whenever the total diet is in excess, (irrespective of any particular food) the power of the diabetic to make use of carbohydrate is reduced. A diabetic should *never* overeat.

17. Q. Is sugar normally present in the blood?
A. Yes, it amounts to about 0.10 per cent true glucose (often expressed as 100 mg. per 100 cc. of blood) if the blood is examined before breakfast. After a meal the percentage increases to about 0.14 (140 mg.) per cent, but drops to normal within approximately two hours. If it rises above 0.15 (150 mg.) per cent in the blood, sugar appears in the urine. The total sugar in the circulating blood is astonishingly little—about 5 grams, or one teaspoonful and there is in the whole body only about half a pound of carbohydrate.

18. Q. Why is the blood tested for sugar if the urine is known to be sugar-free?
A. The diagnosis of diabetes and the results of a faulty diet can be detected earlier in the blood than in the urine. The diet should not be increased unless the

blood sugar is normal. In rare cases the sugar in the blood is normal and yet sugar is present in the urine. These are not true cases of diabetes, but are known as examples of renal glycosuria. In exceptional cases the sugar in the blood may rise above 0.15 (150 mg.) per cent without any sugar in the urine. Rarely there is an individual who constantly has sugar in the urine which is not glucose (grape sugar). This sugar may be pentose or levulose and is harmless. I have recognized about 10 such patients among over 50,000. A nursing mother has milk sugar (lactose) in the urine and this is also harmless.

19. Q. How does the diabetic diet differ from the normal diet?

A. Very little if the diabetes is mild or the patient takes insulin or blood-sugar reducing pills; otherwise, by containing a little less carbohydrate and a little more protein and fat.

20. Q. How much food does a diabetic need?

A. Sufficient for health and strength and, if a child, for growth. This amounts in terms of heat units, calories, to about 20 to 30 calories per kilogram body weight or 10 to 14 calories per pound, but for a child much more, even twice as much, and for a baby three times as much.

21. Q. What is a calorie?

A. A calorie is a unit of heat. It represents the amount of heat which is required to raise 1 kilogram of water 1 degree Centigrade, or approximately 1 pound of water 4 degrees Fahrenheit. All of us need food calories to supply us with warmth and energy, just as a steam boiler requires coal calories and burns these to furnish warmth and energy. We differ from the steam boiler, first, in that we burn our calories very slowly and without a flame and, second, we have (food) calories built into and stored in our living bodies and can live on these if we do not have food, although we get pretty hungry and cross doing so and the sugar in our blood may drop as low as it does from an overdose of insulin.

22. Q. How many calories (heat units) are produced in the body when it uses up 1 gram* of carbohydrate, protein and fat?

A. One gram carbohydrate produces 4 calories; 1 gram protein 4 calories; 1 gram fat 9 calories; 1 gram alcohol 7 calories.

23. Q. How is the treatment of diabetes begun, sugar lowered in the blood and the urine made sugar-free?

A. In mild cases, particularly those who are overweight, by eating less and exercising more; in moderate and severe cases by still greater reduction in the total diet with especial decrease in carbohydrate, and if the urine does not become sugar-free, by the use of insulin or oral drugs. For an average diet, see page 62, Table 2.

24. Q. When the urine becomes sugar free, what next?

A. If more food is needed, the diet is gradually increased, first, in carbohydrate, next in protein and fat, meanwhile testing the urine daily to determine whether the total quantity of food and the different varieties of it are tolerated without the return of sugar in the urine or excess of sugar in the blood. Experienced physicians in the past have insisted upon maintaining the urine sugar free for a month or more before increasing the diet.

*A gram is a small weight. A nickle weighs 5 grams and so does a lump of sugar of full size. One ounce equals 30 grams.

25. Q. How does insulin help?

A. Insulin allows the patient to eat sufficient food to maintain health, strength and growth and be like a normal individual. If he does not manufacture enough insulin in his own pancreas, then he must secure it elsewhere. One unit of insulin "burns up" 1 to 2 grams, and occasionally more, of carbohydrate. If a patient keeps his urine sugar-free and his blood sugar normal with diet or a combination of diet and insulin or drugs, the danger of acidosis (diabetic coma) disappears.

26. Q. What are the "quick", "slow", and "intermediate" insulins?

A. Protamine zinc insulin slowly lowers the blood sugar and its effect lasts for a period of twenty-four to forty-eight hours. The intermediate insulins, NPH, Lente and Globin, act more rapidly and the effect persists twenty-four or twenty hours. Regular or crystalline insulin quickly lowers the blood sugar and the effect lasts six to eight hours.

27. Q. When should insulin be taken?

A. Ten to thirty minutes before a meal.

28. Q. How sterilize the needle and syringe before using?

A. By boiling for five minutes or by keeping them in 70 per cent alcohol or isopropyl alcohol.

29. Q. How measure the insulin?

A. If the syringe holds 1 cubic centimeter and is divided in tenths, each space equals one-tenth of the number of units in the cubic centimeter. If using U-40 insulin, each space equals 1/10 of 40 units or 4 units. If the syringe is graduated for U40 or U80 insulin, the number of units can be read directly on the scale. *Be sure you know the strength of insulin you inject.*

4

30. Q.   Why change site of injection daily?

A.   To prevent poor absorption, abscesses, insulin atrophy and insulin lumps.

31. Q.   If a needle breaks during injection?

A.   Circle the spot where the needle was inserted with ink or other means; draw an arrow showing which way the needle was pointed, then report to your doctor. X-ray the area from two angles because needles are hard to locate. Don't worry. No need for haste.

32. Q.   What is the dose of insulin?

A.   It varies with each case. A patient requires sufficient units to keep his urine sugar-free, his blood sugar normal, enjoy a reasonably varied diet and enough of it to maintain vigor and a suitable body weight. During diabetic coma and in the presence of fever insulin acts less well and more units are required, but when given in sufficient quantity it is life-saving. Exercise lowers the need for insulin.

33. Q.   If one begins the use of insulin, must it be continued indefinitely?

A.   Not in some milder cases. It is dangerous to omit insulin if sugar is present in the urine. When this rule is not followed, diabetic coma may result. Even if the patient does not take food, he should continue the insulin, adding the quick-acting regular or crystalline insulin, (in small and frequent doses during the day) provided the urine shows sugar. If deprived of insulin, cut the diet in half, and avoid exercise so as to reduce the need for calories—your own calories. Never be like one of the foolish virgins. Keep a reserve of insulin, needles and syringes on hand.

34. Q.   What is an insulin reaction?

A. If too much insulin is given, the blood sugar falls below normal and a "reaction" occurs. (*a*) The symptoms of a reaction are hunger, tremor, sweating, unconsciousness. Other symptoms are weakness, pallor, faintness, nervousness, dizziness, dilated pupils, double vision, emotional upsets. Nausea and headache are apt to occur if the reaction is due to protamine insulin. A reaction caused by any kind of insulin may progress to unconsciousness and convulsions. If the sugar in the blood falls suddenly or to a low level, 0.05 per cent or 50 milligrams, symptoms of an insulin reaction occur. They are similar to what one experiences after severe exertion, such as the Marathon run or may be due to lack of food—such as waiting around for someone who is late for dinner. Undoubtedly, such a group of symptoms might appear if these people, in a fasting state, went through severe muscular exertion, like religious fanatics, and fell into a trance.

The urine is free from sugar at the time of a reaction unless it has been collecting in the bladder; then it may contain sugar; a second specimen passed a little later, freshly secreted by the kidneys while the blood is coursing through them has a lower level of sugar, and would be sugar-free. (See Fig. 15, page 139.) Such a specimen is much more comparable with the blood.

An insulin reaction is the result of lowering of sugar in the blood below the normal level. It may occur: (1) if the dose of insulin is not followed soon, (*a*) by food, (*b*) by food containing sufficient carbohydrate, or (*c*) if the digestion is upset and the food is not absorbed, is vomited or lost by diarrhea; (2) as a result of unusual exercise, because exercise lowers the blood sugar; finally, (3) because the diabetes has improved.

The prevention of an insulin reaction is accomplished by regularity for meal hours, avoidance of sudden changes in diet, insulin or exercise and by the use of lunches between meals, especially when long-acting insulins are used.*

Regular insulin must always be followed by food, preferably within thirty minutes and in a *shorter* period if a quick and slowly-acting insulin are taken together. Following regular or crystalline insulin the interval of time before the onset of a reaction is relatively short, but after protamine insulin it is relatively long and may not occur for twenty-four hours. A reaction due to regular or crystalline insulin is more apt to occur in the daytime; one from protamine insulin in the nighttime or on rising in the morning; and from NPH, Globin and Lente insulin in the afternoon. If as much as 5 grams carbohydrate are taken hourly on the hour probably a reaction would seldom occur, or if it did then one might need to change to 10, 15 or 20 grams carbohydrate hourly.

The treatment of an insulin reaction is simple. Raise the lowered blood sugar to a normal level by giving carbohydrate, such as a few lumps of sugar, Karo syrup, orange juice, gingar ale or any form of carbohydrate. If recovery is not prompt, go to a hospital because it may be necessary to give glucose intravenously. Avoid delay.

35. Q. What can a diabetic patient do for himself besides keeping the urine sugar-free.

A. Be cheerful and also be thankful that his disease, instead of being of a hopeless character, is one which his brains will help him to control. He should keep his temper under restraint and not be a spoiled child or pretend to be nervous, but gain the respect of his associates. He should avoid people with colds in the

---

*One patient, whose job involves intricate work with machinery, sleeps eight hours and takes four meals in the remaining sixteen hours; thus he is never long without food in the active part of the day.

head and sore throats; secure a daily action of the bowels; sleep eight to nine hours at night; take time for complete relaxation; and insert exercise into the routine of the forenoon, afternoon and evening.

36. Q. How help prevent diabetes in relatives and friends?

A. First by explaining the dangers of overweight particularly above the age of thirty and telling simple ways to reduce it such as: (1) Leave the table a little hungry; no "seconds." (2) Satisfy the stomach with low-value 3 per cent vegetables instead of with bread and butter. (3) Omit lunches, candy and sodas between meals. Avoid all fat meats and fish, cheese and oil or nuts. Replace pies and pastry with fruit for dessert. (4) Use milk, even skimmed, instead of cream. (5) Encourage exercise. (6) Weigh weekly. (7) By cautioning against the transmission of the disease. Diabetes is hereditary. Two diabetics should not marry one another and have children; the disease also may be transmitted if a diabetic marries a non-diabetic in whose family the disease is present.

37. Q. What is diabetic coma?

A. Diabetic coma implies lack of insulin. It is a state of acid poisoning. The fat in the diet or in the body is imperfectly utilized, resulting in more fatty acids being formed than the body can consume. If neglected, this leads to unconsciousness and can even cause death. If the diet is adequate in carbohydrate and protein and these are utilized, then less fat is required for maintenance and no more than the body can burn. A simple test for acid poisoning, due to excess of ketone bodies—acetone, diacetic acid and β-oxybutyric acid can be made with "Acetest" (directions enclosed with package).

38. Q.   What causes diabetic coma—acid poisoning?
A.   Overeating, infections, too little insulin.

39. Q.   What are typical symptoms of diabetic coma?
A.   Gradual onset of weakness, fatigue, nausea and vomiting, pain in abdomen, deep and difficult breathing, and increasing drowsiness leading to unconsciousness.

40. Q.   How can diabetic coma be prevented?
A.   By keeping sugar-free.   Acid poisoning never occurs unless a patient overeats and fails to burn a sufficient amount of carbohydrate.   He may overeat by breaking the diet and overeating food, or he may over-eat by eating his own body, which is what takes place if he has fever, infections, certain forms of goiter, or food is unutilized because of vomiting, diarrhea or lack of insulin.   *Never omit insulin* if the urine contains sugar, because coma is due to lack of insulin.   Diabetic coma is so dangerous and deceptive that *whenever a patient feels ill, "sick," it is safer to consider it acid poisoning* and:

1. Call the doctor and report your test of the urine.
2. Go to bed.
3. Keep warm.
4. Drink slowly not over one cupful of hot liquid every hour—water, tea, coffee, broth, or oatmeal gruel.
5. Take an enema.
6. Get someone to nurse you.
7. Never omit insulin if urine shows sugar.

When the doctor arrives, if he finds diabetic coma present, he may give insulin every half hour or hour, salt solution under the skin or into a vein, protect the heart and perhaps wash out the stomach, and probably send the patient to a hospital.

41. Q. Can a diabetic be operated upon?

A. Yes. Mild diabetics taking little or no insulin and whose regular diet contains 150 or more grams carbohydrate, and who are sugar-free, receive no food or insulin during the six hours before operation. Diabetics of greater severity receive no food or drink for five or more hours before the operation. After the operation insulin may be given every four to eight hours if sugar appears in the urine, but one should not expect the sugar to disappear immediately in all cases, particularly in those with infections. If a solution of glucose is given intravenously disregard the first specimen of urine voided subsequently, because even in a normal individual some of it may escape into the urine. Some doctors give every four hours 16 units if a red Benedict test, 12 units if orange, 8 units if a yellow, 4 units if green and no insulin if blue or sugar free.

$\dfrac{R}{16}$	$\dfrac{Or}{12}$	$\dfrac{Y}{8}$	$\dfrac{G}{4}$	$\dfrac{B}{0}$

Dr. Marble's method in preparing a patient for operation: Omit all food and drink for 5 or 6 hours before operation. Give half the usual dose of insulin and 1000 cc. normal salt solution containing 100 grams glucose intravenously. Disregard first urine voided because that will contain sugar. Then give insulin as indicated every 4 hours.

RULES BEFORE DISCHARGE FROM HOSPITAL.

Before discharge from the hospital a patient should know how:

1. To test the urine for sugar.
2. To record the diet.
3. To explain the quantity in carbohydrate, protein and fat in the diet.

4. To measure out the prescribed dose of insulin and know when and where to inject it.
5. To describe what to do if sugar returns.
6. To describe what to do if ill, or coma suspected.
7. To describe an insulin reaction—symptoms, cause, prevention and treatment.
8. To state the dangers of (*a*) too much insulin, or (*b*) its total omission (pp. 51 and 54).
9. To care for the feet and explain the reason why.
10. To secure a diabetic identification card signed by patient and physician.

42. Q.　How to avoid complications of diabetes?
A.　Always control the disease daily with diet, exercise, insulin and by tests of the urine. A monthly visit to the physician is advisable the first year and later several times yearly.

5

DIABETIC ARITHMETIC

"And I said of medicine, that this is an art which considers the
constitution of the patient, and has principles of action and reasons
in each case." PLATO: GORGIAS.*

Introduction

A PATIENT can be treated for diabetes successfully
even though he does not know what a calorie is, what
a gram represents or the meaning of the words carbohydrate, protein and fat.   Indeed, some of my patients
cannot read or write.   But I think if one has a disease
it is more fun to know something about it and, as that
Grecian philosopher said years ago, to have "principles
of action and reasons in each case."

R. D. Lawrence, a leading diabetes clinician and the
foremost diabetic now living, writes: ". . . At the beginning of treatment, except in the mildest cases, I
consider it essential that the food should be weighed
out or measured, and this is especially important in
insulin cases," . . . "it is probably wisest to continue to
weigh concentrated carbohydrate foods, such as bread,
toast, fruits, etc.   In any case, every insulin patient
should weigh the food for a few meals every now and
again to make sure that he is keeping close to his diet,
and that the judgment of his eye is not wrong.   I find
this necessary in my own case." . . . "Correct diet is
more important to a diabetic than change of air and
scenery."

*This was the motto Sir William Osler in 1892 placed as an intro-
duction to his first edition of *Principles and Practice of Medicine.*

(57)

It is far simpler in estimating the diet to use the metric than the avoirdupois system. Unfortunately, the more general employment of scales registering pounds and ounces makes this at times difficult. For this reason it is well to know both the metric and avoirdupois systems and to be able to convert the one into the other. The essential values are given in Table 1.

The unit of weight in the metric system is a gram. It is easy to visualize the value of a gram when it is known that a nickel, five-cent coin, weighs exactly 5 grams, a dime about 2.5 grams. A kilogram (1000 grams) is equivalent to 2.2 pounds. Kilograms become more homelike when one's own weight is changed into kilograms. Thus a weight of 132 pounds $(\frac{132}{2.2})=$ 60 kilograms. When computing diets one is guided by weight without clothes (clothes do not require food).

TABLE 1.—THE METRIC AND AVOIRDUPOIS SYSTEMS COMPARED
DRY MEASURE

30 grams = 1 ounce[1]   :   16 ounces = 1.0 pound
1000 grams = 1 kilogram   :   = 2.2 pounds

LIQUID MEASURE

30 cubic centimeters = 1 fluidounce[2] : 32 ounces = 1 quart
1000 cubic centimeters = 1 liter

CALORIES

1 gram carbohydrate = 4 Calories
1 gram protein   = 4 Calories
1 gram fat   = 9 Calories

[1]Actually 28.4 grams.   [2]Actually 29.6 grams

The unit of volume in liquid measure in the metric system is the cubic centimeter. A cubic centimeter of water weighs 1 gram. Thirty cubic centimeters (actually 29.6) make a fluidounce, which is approximately equal to 2 tablespoonfuls of water. One thousand cubic

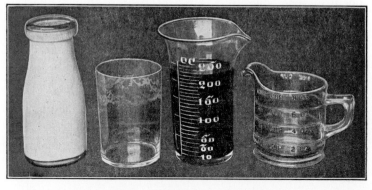

a   *b*   *c*   *d*

FIG. 6.—*a*, milk, ½ pint or 240 cubic centimeters (cc.); *b*, drinking glass, capacity 8 ounces; *c*, 250 cubic centimeters (cc.) graduate; *d*, measuring cup, capacity 8 ounces.

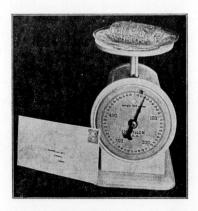

FIG. 7.—Food scales weighing 500 grams.[1] The pointer is at 30 grams which is the equivalent of 1 ounce. I believe in scales, even if they are used for a short time. Without an occasional recourse to scales a patient gets careless.

[1]Convenient food scales of 500 grams' capacity with movable dial are made by John Chatillon & Sons, 89 Cliff Street, New York City.

centimeters, (one liter), are a little more than a quart. One quart (32 ounces) × 30 cc. = 960 cc. (actually 947 cc.) Consider a quart 1000 cubic centimeters or grams. Then, if a patient has 6 per cent sugar and the urine amounts to 4 quarts in 24 hours, he would lose in the urine 4 quarts × 6 per cent (4000 × .06) = 240 grams or approximately ½ pound.

It is worth while to measure the mixed 24-hour quantity of urine every day until treatment is established, because single specimens vary greatly depending upon whether obtained before, between or just after meals.

In estimating carbohydrate, protein and fat in the diet, or sugar in the urine, enough accuracy is obtained in clinical work by considering that 30 grams (gm.) or 30 cubic centimeters (cc.) equal an ounce, dry or liquid measure.

Nearly all the foods upon which diabetic patients live are printed in Tables 3, 4 and 5.[1] Most of the foods in Table 3 come under the head of 3 per cent vegetables. By this is meant that not over 3 per cent (or 3 grams in each 100 grams) of these vegetables may be counted as carbohydrate. As a matter of fact, lettuce, at the beginning of the first column, contains 2.2 per cent, and snap beans, toward the bottom of the second column, occasionally contain as much as 6 per cent carbohydrate. The average percentage of carbohydrate for the entire group would be about 3 per cent, or 1 gram carbohydrate for each 30 grams (1 ounce) of vegetables.

A large saucerful of a 3 per cent vegetable weighs about 150 grams and contains about 5 grams of carbohydrate. Another reason for reckoning these so-called 3 per cent vegetables at 3 per cent available carbohydrate is that when they are cooked considerable carbohydrate is lost in the water used in the cooking. Furthermore, although the carbohydrate may be more

[1] For one day's diet see Table 2, p. 62.

than 3 per cent, we humans, unlike herbivorous animals, cannot assimilate it. This also applies to vegetables in the 6 per cent column. A mixture of 4 portions of 3 per cent and 6 per cent vegetables can be estimated arbitrarily at carbohydrate 20 grams and protein 6

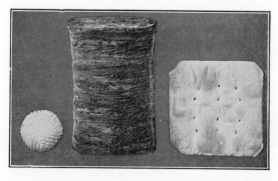

FIG. 8

Butter, 10 grams	Shredded wheat, 30 grams[1]	Uneeda Biscuit,[1] 6 grams[1]
Fat, 8 grams	Carbohydrate, 23 grams	Carbohydrate, 5 grams

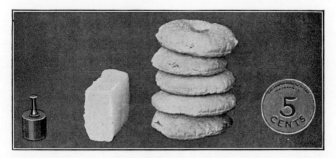

FIG. 9

5-gram weight   Lump sugar, 5 grams   5 oyster crackers, 5 grams
5-cent piece, 5 grams

[1] Original size, now somewhat less, thus illustrating the desirability of weighing foods.

TABLE 2.—A 24-HOUR DIABETIC DIET. ADJUST FOR AGE, SEX AND WEIGHT.[1,2]

Food	Portions	Ounces	Grams	Carbohydrate	Protein	Fat	Calories
Bread	3 lg. slices	3	90	45	8	0	212
Orange	3 medium	15	450	45	0	0	180
3% Vegetables	4 portions	20	600	20	6	0	104
Oatmeal cooked	1 cup	8	240	20	5	2	118
Milk	1½ cups	12	360	18	12	12	228
Egg	1			0	6	6	78
Meat	2 portions	5	150	0	35	25	365
Butter	6 pats	1	30	0	0	25	225
Approximate Total Values:				148	72	70	1500

1 kilogram (kg.) = 2.2 lbs.
30 grams (g.) or cubic
centimeters (cc) = 1 oz.

A patient "at rest"
requires 25 calories per kg.

1 gm. carbohydrate, 4 calories
1 gm. protein, 4 calories
1 gm. fat, 9 calories

[1] Also refer to text page 63 and Tables 3, 4, 5.
[2] Important food Tables 1 to 5, are same as on enclosed yellow card, sold by J. C. Clark Co., 15 Hathaway Street, Boston Massachusetts.

grams, because it is not worthwhile to calculate each separately. In the 20 per cent vegetables almost their full value of carbohydrate is available.

Fruits are arranged in Table 4, p. 66. Their weights in portions which contain 10 or 15 grams of carbohydrate are likewise recorded in grams.

For accuracy shredded wheat, crackers, breads and cereals must be weighed because values are constantly changing. A slice of bread *formerly* weighed 1 ounce but now nearer 25 grams. The carbohydrate in one Matsos is about 25 grams or the equivalent of a slice and a half of bread.

If patients know the food values of the 15 foods mentioned in Table 5, it is seldom more knowledge is required. Patients are advised to buy gram scales but since many households already have ounce scales, Table 2 is so arranged that the quantities of carbohydrate, protein and fat in an ounce (30 grams) of food are placed opposite that food. In Chapter 32 are given the actual percentage values for carbohydrate, protein, and fat in many foods.

FROM FOODS BELOW ADD CARBOHYDRATE, PROTEIN OR FAT
TO DIET—TABLE 2, PAGE 62—AS DESIRED

Food	Ounce	Grams	C.	P.	F.
Bread, 1 slice	1	30	15	3	0
Oatmeal, 1 portion	1	30	20	5	2
Potato, the size of an egg	2	60	12	2	0
Milk	1	30	1.5	1	1
Cream, 20%	1	30	1	1	6
Egg, one			0	6	6
Meat	1	30	0	7	5

This Basic Diet (Table 2, p. 62) can be increased in carbohydrate by the addition of one or more slices of bread, each containing C. 15 grams and P. 2.5 grams, oatmeal, a large portion, C. 20, P. 5, F. 2 grams, biscuits, saltines, Uneedas, graham crackers, each 3–6 grams, and milk for each ounce C. 1.5, P. 1, F. 1 grams. Protein and fat can be added in the form of an egg, P.6, F.6 grams, and cooked meat P.7, F.5 grams, or cheese P.8, F.11 grams per ounce or 30 grams.

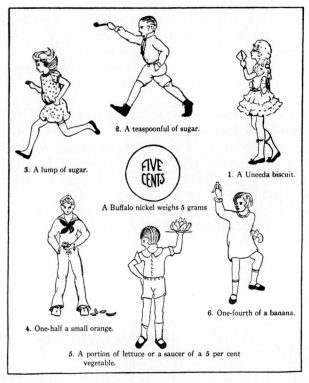

Fig. 10.—A nickel and its equivalents by weight in carbohydrate.

The reason for inserting the food value of uncooked oatmeal instead of cooked oatmeal is due to the variable quantity of water which dry oatmeal takes up during cooking. There is far less difference in the weights of preparations of uncooked oatmeal.

The division of the diet of an adult weighing 110 pounds (50 kilograms) is given in Table 2, p. 62, but the diet is also in part summarized here.

TABLE 3.—FOODS ARRANGED APPROXIMATELY ACCORDING TO CONTENT OF CARBOHYDRATE

Water, clear broths, coffee and tea, can be taken without allowance for food content

Vegetables, Fresh or Canned
Reckon average carbohydrate, utilized, 3%; 6%; 20%

3 per cent		6 per cent	20 per cent
Lettuce	Tomatoes	Turnip	Potatoes
Cucumbers, raw	Radishes	Carrots	Shell Beans
Spinach	Water Cress	Okra	Baked Beans
Asparagus	Snap Beans	Pumpkin	Lima Beans
Celery	Cauliflower	Onions	Corn
Mushrooms	Cabbage	Squash	Boiled Rice
Rhubarb	Egg Plant	Beets	Boiled
Sauerkraut	Broccoli	Green Peas	Macaroni
Endive, raw	Green Peppers.	Brussels Sprouts	
Swiss Chard	Kohl Rabi		
Beet Greens	Kale		
Dandelions	Summer Squash		

Knowing the total quantity of each variety of food eaten by the patient during the day, by using the table of food values (Table 5, p. 67) one can determine the amount of carbohydrate, protein and fat for each given food. Thus 600 grams of 3 per cent vegetables, or 4 cupfuls, were used. Table 5 shows it is assumed that in each cup (150 grams) of 3 per cent vegetables there are 5 grams carbohydrate and 1.5 grams protein and therefore in 600 grams, 4 portions (20 ounces), there would be approximately 20 grams carbohydrate and 6 grams protein. In general, 3 per cent vegetables need not be weighed because they contain so little carbohydrate and fat.

5

TABLE 4.—WEIGHTS OF VARIOUS FRUITS EQUIVALENT TO
10 AND 15 GRAMS OF CARBOHYDRATE

Fruits, Fresh or Canned (Water Packed)

	Weight Equivalent To Carbohydrate	
Fruits	**10 gms.**	**15 gms.**
Grapefruit Pulp............	150 gms.	225 gms.
Strawberries...............	150	225
Watermelon...............	150	225
Cantaloupe...............	150	225
Blackberries...............	120	180
Orange Pulp	**100**	**150**
Pears.....................	90	135
Peaches...................	90	135
Apricots..................	80	120
Raspberries...............	80	120
Plums....................	80	120
Pineapple.................	70	105
Apple....................	70	105
Honeydew Melon..........	70	105
Blueberries...............	70	105
Cherries..................	60	90
Banana...................	50	75
Prunes (cooked)..........	50	75
Ice Cream...............	50	75

A Preliminary Basic Diet

It is easy to prescribe and for a patient to remember this preliminary basic diet: one slice of bread, one orange, ½ cup milk, one egg or a moderate portion of meat, fish or cheese at each meal. During the day, 1 ounce of butter, 4 liberal portions of 3 per cent vegetables. The approximate values in this diet are given in Table 2, p. 62.

TABLE 5.—THE QUANTITY OF CARBOHYDRATE, PROTEIN AND FAT AND THE CALORIC VALUE OF 30 GRAMS (1 OUNCE) OF FOODS IN COMMON USE

30 Grams, 1 oz. Contain Approximately	Carb. C. Gram	Protein P. Gram	Fat F. Gram	Calories
Bread, 1 large slice*..........	15	2.5	0	70
Oatmeal, large portion........	20	5	2	118
Crackers, 2.................	10	1	0	44
Vegetables, 3%, 4 portions....	20	6	0	104
Orange, medium,............	15	0	0	60
Potato.....................	6	1	0	28
Milk......................	1.5	1	1	19
Egg, 1.....................	0	6	6	78
Meat, lean.................	0	7	5	73
Chicken, lean..............	0	8	3	59
Fish, fat-free..............	0	6	0	24
Cheese....................	0	8	10	122
Bacon.....................	0	5	15	155
Cream, 20% light...........	1	1	6	62
Butter.....................	0	0	25	225

*Bread is a great source of worry, because it contains so much carbohydrate and it is so easy to eat an excess of it. Actually, it is said to contain 50 per cent carbohydrate, but when it is dry or toasted the per cent, but not the total quantity of carbohydrate, would be more. The weight of one slice is so variable that the bread should be weighed and half the weight considered to be carbohydrate.

Additions to the diet can be arranged to be made at that meal after which tests for sugar in the urine show the diet already employed has been utilized. The following form which the patient fills out daily at the beginning of treatment, indicates whether the increase in the diet is justified. This form is a valuable method by which to drive home to a patient the results of meals and degree of control of his diabetes. A resort to it occasionally will clear up many obscure conditions.

REPORT OF URINE TESTS

DATE 19	Before breakfast	Before noon meal	Before supper	At bedtime	Insulin			Remarks
					PZI	NPH	RI	
Mo. Day								

The actual percentages of carbohydrate, protein and fat in various other foods are given in the large tables on pages 287–296. From these it is easy to calculate the quantity of carbohydrate, protein and fat in any food which a patient takes when the total quantity of food eaten is known. Patients and nurses are repeatedly confused by such tables, forgetting that if the quantity of carbohydrate in milk is 5 per cent (see page 291), 100 grams of milk (or in this case cubic centimeters) would contain 5 grams of carbohydrate, just as 5 per cent interest on $100 for a year would be $5. Lobster (see page 291) for instance, contains 16 per cent protein, and therefore 100 grams of lobster contain (100×0.16) 16 grams protein. Incidentally, this is a good food on which to lose weight and always an appropriate gift to a diabetic.

The use of percentages, however, is employed far more in determining the quantity of sugar voided in the urine by diabetic patients during the twenty-four hours. If an individual voids 2000 cc. (cubic centimeters) of urine, which can be roughly estimated as 2 quarts, and the percentage of sugar is 6 per cent, it is plain that the quantity of sugar lost in the urine during the twenty-

four hours would be 2000 × 0.06 = 120 grams, or
¼ pound. As a lump of sugar amounts to about 5
grams, this would mean that the equivalent of 24
lumps of sugar was lost in the urine in one day.

"There is nothing which effort and unceasing and diligent care
cannot overcome." (Seneca)

"To *will* is a great thing, dear sisters, for Action and Work
usually follow will, and almost always Work is accompanied by
success. These three things, Will, Work, Success, fill human
existence." (Pasteur[1])

[1] Vallery-Radot: Life of Pasteur, N.Y. McClure Phillips & Co.
p. 15, 1906.

6

EFFICIENCY IN VISITS TO A DOCTOR

ENCOURAGE a complete physical examination from the crown of your head to the soles of your feet. Undress entirely so that it will be possible for the physician to pick up anything wrong. Diabetics live so long that they develop diseases which have no connection with diabetes. Because of frequent visits to a physician signs of these should be detected earlier than in a non-diabetic. Therefore, diabetics should be less likely to die of cancer and tuberculosis than are other people.

A patient frequently fails to gain all he should from a visit to his physician because he does not furnish the facts upon which advice for further treatment should be based. Physical appearance alone is by no means a sufficient guide to the careful doctor. Information ought to be presented concerning tests of the urine, the diet, units of insulin used, or oral drugs, insulin reactions or any other complications.

1. Information Obtained by Examination of the Urine

The physician should know whether the urine of the patient is free from sugar, or, if present, how much it contains. This is essential in order to prescribe insulin, the diet, oral medication or exercise. The patient should therefore, when practical, take with him a specimen of the urine saved from the entire twenty-four hour amount. This is far more difficult to obtain, because now patients are so active in work or play that weekends often furnish the only opportunity available. To collect such a specimen of urine, discard that voided at 7 A.M. and then save all urine passed up to and including that obtained at 7 the next morning. Take 60 cc. (2 ounces) of the thoroughly mixed twenty-four-hour quantity for examination. Record the twenty-four-hour amount of urine, the date and the name on the bottle. The large bottle in which the urine is being collected should be kept in a cool place. It is best to procure for this special purpose a bottle with a tight-fitting cork, sufficiently large to hold the entire twenty-four hour amount of urine. Select a bottle with a large mouth, that it may be more easily cleansed, scalding it out daily. Urine so collected decomposes slowly. On account of the presence of sugar, diabetic urines are prone to ferment, and if fermentation occurs, a portion of the sugar disappears and thus spoils the test. A good preservative is xylol, of which $\frac{1}{2}$ teaspoonful can be placed in a 2-quart bottle before the collection of urine begins.

From the difference between the carbohydrate in the diet and the total quantity of sugar which has escaped in the urine, it is possible to learn how much of the carbohydrate of the diet has been lost. Patients more and more will desire to know how much this is and the percentage lost. Of course, perfection—100 per cent utilization—is to be desired but at times one must be content with 95 or 90 per cent utilization in order to guard against insulin reactions. I regret such a concession.

The use of insulin has emphasized the value of the examination of single specimens of urine. The urine voided before a meal may be free from sugar, while that voided one or two hours after eating may show sugar. This indicates that either the carbohydrate should be reduced at that particular meal or insulin increased. If the urine voided upon arising is not sugar-free, it shows that the diabetes is not controlled and if the patient is using protamine zinc insulin that more of it is required.

At times the urine will contain sugar on rising because it collected in the bladder at some hour during the night. In this event a second specimen voided a little later, representing freshly secreted urine, may be sugar-free. If the bladder is thoroughly emptied and a fresh specimen of the urine voided one-half hour later is tested, the result of this second test will more closely conform to the sugar in the blood and thus indicate the condition of the diabetes for that half hour rather than for the several hours before the first voiding. Unless the urine is sugar-free on rising the patient is handi-capped all day. If the urine shows sugar later in the day, it is a sign that crystalline, regular NPH or a similar insulin should be added, diet altered or more exercise required.

Temporarily it may be desirable to save the day's urine in four portions. The urine voided at about an hour after breakfast may show considerable sugar, but shortly thereafter, or more surely later in the morning, may become sugar-free. If the rising, before supper and retiring specimens are free from sugar the patient can consider himself about perfect.

A convenient method to report specimens is as follows:

Date	Rising	Before Lunch	Before Supper	Retiring
January 1..........	Red	Orange	Yellow	Green
January 2..........	R	Or	Y	G
January 3..........	Y	G	B	B
January 4..........	B	B	B	B

2. Information Obtained by Examination of the Diet

The quality and quantity of the food eaten during the twenty-four hours should be recorded. If thirty min-utes are allowed for the length of a return visit to the physician's office, it is no exaggeration to say that unless this summary of the diet is kept, one-third to one-half of the visit is spent by the physician in learning what the patient has eaten. For this reason patients should always bring a list of what they ate in the preceding twenty-four hours. If the weights are not known, record in portions—the number of slices of bread, portions of fruit, amount of milk, cereal and vegetables.

3. Insulin

An accurate record of the quantity of insulin taken should be furnished. *It is a good plan to show the doctor the syringe and the bottle of insulin used.* It is important to know when the insulin has been taken and how much at a time. Has there been an insulin reaction, and what was the cause, and how can another be prevented? Show the doctor where you inject the insulin at the same time you exhibit your pretty (or at least clean) feet.

4. Information Obtained by Examination of the Blood

The course of treatment of a case of diabetes is also regulated by the quantity of sugar in the blood. If the sugar in the blood can be kept at the normal figure before a meal, 0.1 (100 mg.) per cent and not over 0.15 (150 mg.) true glucose after a meal, the patient should not show sugar in the urine. Formerly, we used the Folin-Wu method of analysis and the upper limit of normal fasting was 120 mg. and after food, 170 mg. It is advantageous to have blood-sugar tests at various times in the day. The blood sugar in health usually reaches its greatest height about one-half hour after a meal, but in diabetics the peak comes later and the curve falls more slowly. The percentage of sugar in the blood usually reaches its lowest limit in the late forenoon. This is the period when the patient taking quick-acting insulin, regular or crystalline, is most exposed to an insulin reaction, but when using Globin, NPH or Lente insulin a reaction is more apt to occur in the late afternoon. The blood sugar with patients doing well with protamine, NPH, Globin or Lente insulin should be at a normal level before breakfast. But remember, a change in the quantity or quality of the diet or amount of exercise may bring on a reaction at any hour. When our patients took calisthenics one evening in the Hospital Teaching Clinic the blood sugar dropped so low that reactions developed. Exercise is most beneficial in the treatment of diabetes.

5. Body Weight

If the patient has scales, the weight before breakfast, preferably undressed, for children the weight and height without shoes, should be taken on the morning of the visit.

6. Heredity

Any new details about heredity should be reported. Only by cooperation between patient and physician will new cases of diabetes in the family be detected and others perhaps prevented. Early recognition and instant beginning of treatment may lessen the severity of the diabetes for a patient's whole lifetime. Unless all our ideas upon heredity are wrong, the million unrecognized diabetics in the country are for the most part relatives of known diabetics and the diabetics should help to find them. The least they can do is to preach against the relative of a diabetic, or in fact anyone, being fat. All women should avoid having big babies, especially by those who have a diabetic relative. The mother of a 12 or 14 pound baby can be expected, eventually, to develop diabetes.

7. Notebook

Start a notebook on the first day of treatment and show it to the physician at each visit. All questions about symptoms and diet which have arisen since the former visit should be set down neatly with space left for an answer to each question. It is a common error

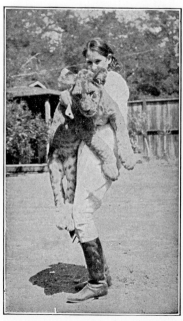

FIG. 11.—Case No. 6999. Age at onset of diabetes eleven years five months in December, 1926. Alive in 1953.

If a diabetic child can control a lion she can certainly control diabetes.

for patients to ask the same question many times, whereas if the answer is written down by the physician the question would thus be answered once for all time.

The notebook should contain a statement as to whether sugar has been present or absent in the urine since the last report to the physician.   Such data can be gathered on one page as in the diagram on page 68. When a patient comes to my office with a single specimen of urine instead of a portion taken from the twenty-four-hour quantity, is confused about the number of units of insulin taken, has no record of the food eaten during the preceding day, and starts in to recount that he had nothing but eggs, meat and fish, then later remembers that he had a little cream and various vegetables, then with prompting recalls butter and an orange and a little oatmeal, potato or bread, I always pity him, and on very exceptional occasions am able to recall with satisfaction, after the interview, Solomon's soliloquy in Proverbs xvi, verse 32.

"He that is slow to anger is better than the mighty; and he that ruleth his spirit than he that taketh a city."

7

EXERCISE ESSENTIAL IN TREATMENT

Work shortens the day, but lengthens the life.

Exercise

THE diabetic should plan to keep his body strong and his mind alert. He has a disease which makes him susceptible to complications, particularly to infections, acute and chronic, general or localized in one part or another of the body, but especially in the lower extremities. He should take advantage of sunlight and fresh air because of the resistance to disease which they promote; he should exercise because in his muscles sugar is burned and thus more carbohydrate may be allowed and less insulin required. Case No. 632 said a game of golf was worth 5 units, and any diabetic mountain climber will tell you how much his diet can be increased and his insulin reduced by a long day's hike. The diabetic who does not utilize exercise in the treatment of his disease is failing to take advantage of its pleasantest remedy; and by exercise I mean working about the house or yard, walking up and down stairs, back and forth to school or work and going outdoors at noontime as well. It is exercise day in and day out which counts rather than an hour or two of play once a week. Bouchardat said: "He should earn his bread by the sweat of his brow."

Dr. Sabine, of Brookline, made the remark, based upon the experience of his many years of general practice, that those of his patients who took active camping trips in the woods bore the stress of modern life best.

By this means exercise was combined with mental relaxation. The good effects of relaxation with exercise last for months. It is only natural to conclude that if the muscles, in which is stored one-half of the carbohydrate of the body, are kept in good condition by training, a favorable effect must be produced upon the general metabolism of carbohydrate.

The effect of increase of exercise upon the well-being of fat diabetics has been pronounced, and it is striking how many miles a semi-ill or obese diabetic patient can learn to walk in two weeks. The patients are encouraged to take their walks soon after meals and to go outdoors several times a day. As a result of exercise the urine becomes sugar free. No case should be considered too far advanced for an attempt at muscular redevelopment.

So important is exercise for the proper assimilation of carbohydrate that even surgical patients are urged to exercise. Occasionally this is accomplished by pulley weights attached to the foot of the bed and by dumbbells, but for others passive exercises or bed gymnastics are recommended. Even for non-diabetic patients, such exercises are now routine immediately after operations. The so-called Buerger exercises (see page 181) may be advantageous almost as much from their effect upon the whole body as upon the lower extremities. This undoubtedly explains in part why diabetic patients today withstand surgical operations better than formerly. A diabetic patient with rheumatism is greatly handicapped. Relieve the rheumatism, begin exercise, and much of the insulin may be omitted.

Exercises for the promotion of the circulation in the legs are of great service. They may ward off gangrene. Such exercises are described on page 181–182.

Case No. 804, (duration 10 yrs.) a patient whose diabetes changed from severe to moderate and finally from moderate to mild under his own care at home, wrote that he considered exercise of the greatest importance. He said that he had the best garden of anyone in his city.

Case No. 7500 (duration 29 years), a young farmer, had an insulin reaction after chopping wood in the forest.

Case No. 352 exceeded the normal life expectancy for his age at the onset of his diabetes and lived 23 years. Throughout this entire time he led a most active existence. Moreover this was accomplished many years before insulin was discovered. He was a pioneer and his case at that early date (1912) was of great value to me in my treatment of other patients. He wrote:

"First, it is very hard to start the exercise, and the less one feels inclined to start it the more one needs it. Second, it is neither necessary nor desirable that the exercise should be violent. I found a quiet ride of an hour, walking or jogging, after taking something on the stomach, started up my old metabolism for the whole day. If I rode hard, I got tired out."

Finally, it is astonishing how much exercise a diabetic in training can take. One of my severe cases, living on a strict diet, several years ago walked between 20 and 30 miles in one day. Exercise of the most strenuous type is borne well if the patient will only adjust his diet and insulin to it. Even in the presence of disease of the kidney I have been amazed at the amount of hard work patients apparently could do.

Athletic contests are allowable for diabetics today, but on account of the danger of a reaction, as a result of the strenuous exercise, every diabetic under such circumstances should have his "buddy" or the trainer keep an alert eye upon him. Insulin reactions are very commonly brought on by exercise, but that is no contraindication. Either the diet can be increased or the insulin reduced.

A letter from Case 1729. Age at onset 18 years in 1918. Living 1959. A 41-year-duration case!

"DEAR DR. JOSLIN:

"I have just returned from a ski trip in the Rocky Mountains and in view of the fact that I am a diabetic it seems worth while to let you know a few of the details. It might serve as a little encouragement to other fellow patients.

"In our party were seven large and hardy individuals each carrying bedding and personal effects as well as some food, the whole pack varying between 20 to 35 pounds. We covered in all 250 miles over passes, through valleys in temperatures as low as minus 17, sleeping in cabins when possible, otherwise making camp in the snow. At times our food ran very low. One day in particular we traveled from 8 A.M. till 9.15 P.M. through deep snow. Our allowance in food eaten (estimated, of course) that day was not more than 2000 calories.

"We were the first persons to penetrate the region (Jasper Park) on skis and the first to reach and ascend in winter the Columbia Icefields, L., who stroked the famous Yale Olympic crew in 1924 S., a Norwegian, and myself.

"It seems like a schoolboy trick to brag about this sort of thing, but as I took a dose of insulin before a roaring campfire, temperature around zero and snowing, the thought occurred to me that it might be perhaps an unique experience for a diabetic to be in, 100 miles from the nearest railroad. It is from this standpoint that I am writing rather than from the standpoint of a Richard Halliburton.

"Sorry to bore you with this. Also, sorry not to have as yet checked on blood sugar and urine. General health and fitness fine.

Sincerely,————————"

I often tell my diabetic classes how the blood-sugar lowering effect of exercise was run across unexpectedly by Dr. Sam Levine, the well-known heart specialist. Like Saul in the Bible (I Samuel ix:3) who went out to seek his father's asses but returned with a kingdom, Sam Levine planned to study the effect of exercise upon the circulation of athletes at the end of the Marathon run of 28 miles. He found the runners weak, trembling, perspiring and verging on lack of mental control. Along with his other tests, he tested their blood sugar and the upshot of the experiment was that he found it as low as in an insulin reaction. So that, like Saul, he returned from his quest with a new and totally unanticipated realm of scientific discovery—a beautiful example of serendipity.

Former President A. Lawrence Lowell of Harvard University described so well in his account of the development of the English Constitution how knowledge progresses unwittingly that I quote his words. "It may be stated of the makers of the British parliamentary government as has been said of Columbus, that when he started on his voyage he did not know where he was going, when he got there he did not know where he was, and when he got back he did not know where he had been; and yet he discovered America. Like his the action was intentional, and in its direct objects perfectly logical, but led naturally to results wholly unexpected. I think, therefore, the example of the British parliamentary system shows that with men, as with animals, a continual conscious adaptation to immediate objects may sometimes, if the conditions are favorable, lead to a fully self-consistent and harmonious system which to the authors is quite unforeseen, and which is not only very different from, but even quite inconsistent with, the theories . . . that they retain continuously throughout the process." (in *Factors Determining Human Behavior*, Harvard University Press, Cambridge, Massachusetts, 1937, pp. 129, 130.)

Exercise, however, is a two-edged sword. For it to be beneficial the individual must have insulin available in his body. A normal man has an abundance of insulin; a mild diabetic has less but yet enough insulin so that he too can benefit by exercise, but a severe diabetic must supplement his supply by injecting insulin, otherwise exercise will do harm. Without it to help him utilize his store of carbohydrate and the little formed from protein, he must fall back upon more fat for nourishment than he can safely burn. A severe diabetic without insulin, with disease uncontrolled may go into a diabetic coma with increased exercise, because he must burn up more fat than the system can tolerate.

6

Insulin, especially protamine insulin, changes a diabetic so nearly to a normal individual that during exercise he utilizes carbohydrate beautifully, but if the carbohydrate is lacking, a low blood sugar and, in consequence, a reaction may develop. The same thing happens with athletes. Therefore, when about to take

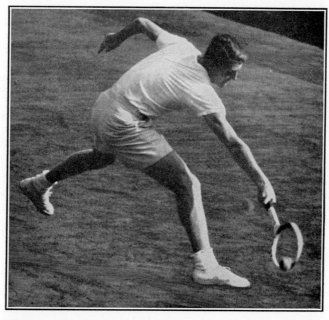

Fig 12.—Hamilton Richardson, Rhodes scholar and champion tennis player, may require a lump of sugar every 20 minutes during a match.

extra and strenuous exercise or during it, the diabetic should eat additional carbohydrates as well as protein and fat.

To many persons exercise seems a luxury, but a diabetic is fortunate in that he can always consider exercise a necessity. Exercise is essential in the treatment of diabetes.

Professor Meythaler of Germany writes, "I have a severe diabetic, a postman, who daily needed 100 units of insulin. His duty was to ride his bicycle 25 kilometers. On account of the danger of hypoglycemia, before he started he would stick his head out the window to see which way the wind blew and when it was against him, he injected 20 units less of insulin."

Rest

Rest is essential. A tired child is put to bed and wakens refreshed; two of the most noted surgeons in the country, the Mayo brothers, were not ashamed to leave their guests at the table and lie down for fifteen minutes after their luncheon; the best treatment for a failing heart is to put its owner in bed for a week or a month. Diabetic patients should rest often, should never allow themselves to get overtired. The diet is designed to give a rest to the pancreas. Sleep nine hours and more if you can. Short periods of complete relaxation yield maximal returns. It is astonishing how much a ten-minute rest will lower a high blood pressure.

Mental Attitude

Do not forget you have diabetes but do not talk about it. Mental diversion is desirable. The cultivation of imperturbability, so greatly advocated by Sir William Osler and his prototype, Sir Thomas Browne, will help a diabetic even more than a nondiabetic.

The man who has a job is the happy man, and as a rule the harder a man works the happier he is and the less bother he is to the other members of his family.

At one time I feared the effect of emotional upsets upon the diabetic, but the longer I treat diabetics the less importance do I assign to mental perturbations. Life near the front in France in 1918 taught me worries did not cause diabetes or make it worse.

The art of learning how to get the most out of life under all circumstances must be cultivated by any patient. It takes time, though, and practice to accommodate one's methods of living to changed conditions, but it pays to study the problem.

My neighbor in Oxford, Massachusetts, Mr. Alfred M. Chaffee, often said, "Make your work your play and your play your work."

Success in Treatment

Never forget that if you make a success of your own case, you are aiding some other diabetic and indirectly helping all diabetics to secure or retain their jobs. And, furthermore, each diabetic who wins a prize protects and advances the reputation of the whole group. Unfortunately the reverse is also true. A diabetic who disregards universally approved diabetic laws or traffic rules assumes a grave responsibility.

The first patient to receive insulin in Toronto was in 1922; our first case, August 7, 1922, but insulin did not become generally available until 1923, so that until 1963 the number of diabetics with a duration of forty years or more will be few, but in 1938 we had at least forty-eight. The average duration of life since onset of diabetes of our 85 Quarter Century Victory Medal cases is 33 years. Fortunate they are if they can leave this world at the height of their activity as described by Homer in the Odyssey when he recorded the first coronary thrombosis in literature, "and Phoebus Apollo shed his gentle darts upon Phrontis, the son of Oneta, Menelaus' helmsman, and he dropped dead with the steering oar of the moving ship within his hands." (Homer: Odyssey—c 900 B.C.)

8

THE DIET OF NORMAL INDIVIDUALS

Food and Fuel

Food is fuel for the body, just as gasoline is fuel (food) for an automobile. Man and automobile depend upon fuel as a source of energy. In case the gasoline gives out the automobile will stop, but if the food gives out the man will not immediately die, because he carries a good deal of his fuel around with him stored up in his body, chiefly as fat, a lesser amount as protein in the muscles and tissues and, third, a very little as carbohydrate, animal starch (glycogen) and sugar. This is found in the liver and muscles, with a trifling amount in the blood, organs and tissues.

A fasting man at the Carnegie Nutrition Laboratory in Boston went without food for thirty-one days, living upon his reserve supply of food, in other words his own tissues. He used up about all his carbohydrate in five days and then depended upon his own fat and protein. During this period he lost 29 pounds.

Just as one can measure how much gasoline is required for an automobile to run 100 miles, so one can measure how much food is necessary for a man to live for twenty-four hours and do a given amount of work. Small automobiles require less gasoline than large automobiles, and this is pretty much true of individuals, for the food which they need depends upon their weight. There are exceptions. Children require proportionately more food, because they are growing and more active, and old people require less, because they have ceased to grow and are quieter. If an adult eats like a child,

he will grow fat.   How unfortunate it is that there is
no one to spank him and thus save him from acquiring
diabetes later; however, indigestion occasionally comes
to the rescue.   Just as the automobile depends upon
gasoline, oil and water, the human automobile depends
upon carbohydrate, protein and fat, water, various salts
and vitamins.   If the food value of 1 gram ($\frac{1}{30}$ of an
ounce) of each of the foods, carbohydrate, protein and
fat is known, and also the quantities of these that are
eaten, the total food value of the diet can be determined
and one can calculate how much it is necessary to have
to live, just as one can calculate how many miles an
automobile can run on a gallon of gasoline.   The nutritive value of the diet is readily computed.   See Tables
2, 3, 4, 5, pages 62, 65, 66, 67.

Another method allows the food required by a given
individual to be calculated far more accurately.   By
this method one can determine the oxygen consumed
and carbon dioxide given off in a specified period of time
and thereby calculate the heat set free.   If this is done
twelve hours after food is eaten and while one is at rest,
it is termed the basal metabolism.   Patients with certain
diseases of the thyroid gland have a high metabolism
and others have a low metabolism.   Thus, they are said
to be burning up their body tissue; more rapidly or
more slowly than normal individuals.   Consequently,
they are apt to be thin or fat.   The metabolism of diabetics when properly treated should be normal.   When
we overfed them it was high, but when we underfed
them at Dr. F. M. Allen's suggestion, it was low and
they lived longer.

This total heat represents energy which has been derived from the oxidation (burning up or utilization) of
the three foodstuffs—carbohydrate, protein and fat.   It
is unessential whether the foodstuffs oxidized have been
taken within a few moments as food or whether they
represent food deposited in the body as fat (fat tissue),

protein (muscle tissue) or carbohydrate (glycogen, *i.e.*, animal starch). Knowing the total heat given off, it is not a difficult matter to calculate how much carbohydrate, protein and fat were burned to produce it. Experiments have shown that the heat which is liberated in the body from the burning of 1 gram of protein or of carbohydrate produces 4 calories, from 1 gram of fat 9 calories and from 1 gram of alcohol 7 calories. Fat, as would be expected, is more than twice as nourishing as carbohydrate or protein.

The needs of the body for fuel vary not only from day to day and hour to hour, but from moment to moment. The calories required by the average normal adult for the twenty-four hours when at rest are about 25 per kilogram (2.2 pounds), or 11 per pound, body weight. If the individual is sitting in a chair instead of lying on a couch 20 per cent more energy is required. Too often in dietetic computations it is assumed that the caloric needs of the body can be accurately estimated. As a matter of fact, the error in such computations is considerable. The reason for this is apparent if one observes the attitudes and motions of individuals. The one is quiet, the other restless; the one avoids exertion, the other is all activity. In disease these differences of habit and disposition are accentuated. A diabetic patient, Case No. 1541, a woman, aged fifty-eight years, confined for a year to her bed with paralysis, remained sugar-free, held her weight constant and the diet, accurately weighed by a trained nurse for the entire period, averaged 20 calories per kilogram per twenty-four hours.

I learned from my friend, Professor Benedict, that the expenditure of 1 calorie of heat is required to rise from a sitting position in front of a door, turn the key in the door, and sit down. A single 65-watt electric light bulb gives off approximately 45 calories per hour, which represents a little less than the heat, (basal metabolism) of an adult weighing 50 kilograms (110 pounds).

Various concrete examples of what calories derived from food will enable an individual to do are here given. To walk one hour on a level road at the rate of 2.7 miles an hour requires 160 calories *above* that of keeping quiet (Lusk). I suspect one will not err greatly if for each mile of walking one allows 1 calorie per 1 kilogram body weight. A man of 60 kilograms (132 pounds) walking up one flight of stairs, 10 feet high, expends about 3 calories.

Sewing and knitting require about 9 calories, typing at the rate of 50 words a minute 30 calories per hour more than that for the same subject sitting quietly in a chair, but washing, sweeping and scrubbing floors require 50 calories additional. Ironing and dish-washing each require about 25 calories additional.

One forgets that an individual doing heavy work does not require additional calories for the entire twenty-four hours. With the cessation of work the need falls abruptly. Furthermore, the actual period of heavy work is short and represented by minutes rather than hours. If of a pessimistic nature one has only to watch street laborers, though a far more enjoyable and as scientific a proof is furnished by the minutes spent in actual play by football teams. In one entire game the minutes in which the ball was actually in play numbered only eleven instead of sixty. As age advances less calories are required and a woman above the age of sixty-six years, will have a twenty-four hour-heat production of about 1000 calories when in a state of complete rest. It is cheaper to board an old man than a young boy.

The diet of normal and diabetic individuals differs very little these days, chiefly because of the discovery of insulin. At one time my hospital patients did not have over 31 grams of carbohydrates per day. Today, few patients have less than 150 grams of carbohydrate, or the *equivalent* of 10 tablespoonfuls of sugar or 10 slices of bread. Insulin is not wholly responsible for this. We have learned that if we do not overfeed a patient, then his ability to get the full benefit of the carbohydrate in his diet increases. Consequently, all are careful about the total food allowed, and no longer reduce the carbohydrate to a minimum and raise the fat to a maximum.

Composition of the Normal Diet

The ordinary diet for a man, weight 132 pounds, (60 kilograms) at office work contains about 250 grams of carbohydrate, 75 grams of protein and 60 grams of fat. This would amount to 1840 calories in the twenty-four hours, or about 31 calories per kilogram.

The quantity of protein in the normal diet of an adult is decidedly less than 100 grams. It is safe for an individual to live upon 1 gram protein per day for *each* kilogram body weight. Protein is animal food to a large degree; hence its high cost; carbohydrate comes from the vegetable kingdom and is therefore cheap. If an excess of protein is burned the other foods are also consumed more rapidly—and there is more chance of the heat so produced to go to waste. Old people often eat too little rather than too much protein.

The quantity of fat in the normal diet varies partly from choice and partly from economic reasons. In general in those cases in which the carbohydrate in the diet is high the fat is low, and *vice versa*.

The more agreeable varieties of fat, such as butter, cream, bacon and oil, are expensive foods, but oleomargarine can be substituted safely for butter. Fat is also a concentrated food, not only because it has twice the caloric value of either carbohydrate or protein, but because it occurs more frequently in pure form. Oil, butter and lard contain little water, whereas except for pure sugar and starch most carbohydrates and proteins are diluted five to ten times with water. The body itself is about three-fifths water.

Today much is said about the danger of bringing on arteriosclerosis, or hardening of the arteries, by eating too much fat, particularly animal fats and milk fats instead of vegetable fats. Diabetics should proceed slowly. It is possible the saturated solid animal fats are more likely to produce atherosclerosis and an increase of cholesterol than the unsaturated, liquid vegetable fats, *e.g.* corn oil, but the nutritionists of the country, in a recent session did not feel warranted in radically changing the diet of the average American.

At present we have no proof that the radical reduction of animal fats and their replacement with vegetable fats has prolonged the duration of life for the diabetic.

The chief source of error in calculating the total caloric value of the diet, and especially of the diabetic diets, is in the estimation of fat. I am very skeptical about the accuracy of the so-called high-carbohydrate low-fat diets in which the fat is supposed to be 50 grams or less. Anyone can realize this upon examining a piece of meat with its fringe of fat. The fat in bacon is most variable, and in amount its value can only be approximately estimated. Portions of bacon, I found, lost from 43 to 67 per cent of fat in the cooking. For this reason my patients are taught to weigh their bacon after it is cooked.

Eggs contain approximately 6 grams of protein and 6 grams of fat. How gross our caloric reckonings are is obvious if a collection of eggs is weighed. The weight of the heaviest egg in a collection of 56 eggs was 72 per cent more than that of the lightest. The 6 grams of protein are equally divided between the white and the yolk, but the 6 grams of fat are all in the yolk. One egg contains between $\frac{1}{4}$ and $\frac{1}{2}$ gram of cholesterol.

Milk and cream are desirable in the treatment of

diabetes, but they must be prescribed and taken with care because of the large quantity of carbohydrate, protein and fat which they represent. Milk also is valuable because it contains calcium (lime), which is necessary for the bones. A glass of milk, 240 grams or cubic centimeters (8 ounces), is drunk so easily that one is apt to forget that it contains 12 grams carbohydrate, 8 grams protein and 8 grams fat. Thirty cubic centimeters (1 ounce) of whole milk, skimmed milk or buttermilk contain 1.5 grams of carbohydrate and 1 gram of protein. Whey contains 5 per cent carbohydrate, but practically no proteins or fat. Cream and koumiss contain about 3 per cent carbohydrate, or 1 gram to the ounce. The Jewish sour cream contains about one-half as much. With the discovery of insulin the need for the diabetic to take an excess of fat vanished, but by no means should we fail to take advantage of its nutritive value.

Cream, butter and cheese are high in nutritive value because they contain so much fat. They must be greatly restricted or even eliminated if a patient desires to live on a low-fat diet or to lose weight. Cheese made from skimmed milk theoretically would be practically free from fat, but actually may contain as much as 15 per cent. The high-protein value of milk—1 gram to the ounce, 32 grams to the quart—is important to consider, not alone because of the protein itself, but also because from protein sugar is formed.

Vitamins

Fortunately, the diabetic diet is adequate in vitamins. To be on the safe side, there is no harm in taking one standard polyvitamin—a mixture of all vitamins—daily. Such can be purchased at about half price if the name of the maker is not specified. It is now also common knowledge that certain food constituents other than protein, carbohydrate, fat and minerals are essential for proper growth and development of the body and for the maintenance of a proper state of nutrition and health. Advances in our knowledge of these food substances, called vitamins, have been made so rapidly in the last several years that any account is almost certain to be out-of-date within a short time. Unfortunately, there is no ready test for an individual's needs for vitamins. If there were, millions of dollars would be saved.

1. *Vitamin A*

Source: butter, egg yolk, carrots, and to a less extent leaves of food plants. The green vegetables and carrots contain no vitamin A, but do contain carotene transferable in part into vitamin A by the liver; it is readily stored, thus accounting for its presence in halibut- and codliver oil. The liver of diabetics may have difficulty in converting carotene into vitamin A. In such cases the skin may take on a yellowish tinge, particularly in the palms and soles, suggesting jaundice. Milk and eggs contain both carotene and vitamin A. Spinach ranks first in richness of vitamin A; carrots and liver come next, followed by cream cheese and native lettuce. The content of cod- and halibut-liver oil varies with the sample.

Lack of vitamin A in animals leads to decreased appetite and decreased growth, may interfere with reproduction and lactation, brings on xerophthalmia and certain types of night blindness. It is one of the vitamins whose adequate supply may lead to prevention of certain types of infections.

2. *Vitamin B Complex*

This is made up of at least twelve factors, of which thiamin, riboflavin and niacin are the most prominent members.

(a)   *Thiamin, vitamin B_1*

Source: Found chiefly in whole-grain cereals, yeast, legumes, nuts, liver, less in eggs, meat, especially pork, and milk, in which it is more or less combined with phosphorus. In refined cereals thiamin is negligible. Today white breads are customarily enriched with vitamins so that from this standpoint it makes no difference whether wheat or whole-grain bread is eaten. A century ago, before the refinement of grains, it is said our ancestors had ten times as many vitamins as we have.

Deficiency of thiamin leads to beri-beri and polyneuritis in animals, retarded growth just as with vitamin A, and in man deficiency may lead to loss of appetite, peripheral neuritis and cardiovascular symptoms. It is important during pregnancy and lactation. It is especially needful in patients who are fed subcutaneously or intravenously, and a relapse of symptoms may occur following glucose and salt infusions. Loss of appetite is usually the first symptom of thiamin deficiency, and appetite may return within twenty-four hours following its administration. *In general, if treatment of any type of deficiency in vitamins is not effective within one month, the diagnosis must be reviewed.*

The value of thiamin chloride in the treatment of the neuritis accompanying pellagra is remarkable, and it acts somewhat similarly in alcoholic neuritis but, unfortunately, massive doses of even 50,000 I.U. daily act very slowly if at all in the relief of diabetic neuritis.

When thiamin is deficient, the products of carbohydrate metabolism, namely, pyruvic acid, accumulate in the blood and tissues. Give thiamin and this is remedied. Thiamin may also be instrumental in the formation of fat from carbohydrate. The higher the carbohydrate of the diet the greater the need for vitamin B_1.

(b) Riboflavin, Vitamin B_2

Source: liver, yeast and milk, meat, eggs and leafy vegetables. Milk, cream, cheese and ice cream provide the main source of riboflavin. Lack of it leads to loss of appetite, aversion for food, and cessation of growth, loss of hair, maceration and transverse fissures of the lips and at the corners of the mouth, and a thickened, pale, gelatin-looking tongue.

(c)   Niacin

Source: similar to that of thiamin, especially liver, brown rice, yeast, particularly brewer's yeast, meat, milk, eggs and green, leafy vegetables. It is nearly specific in the prevention and treatment of pellagra. Its deficiency may be associated with stomatitis, and swollen, sore and scalloped, indented tongue for some time preceding its red character.

The importance of niacin and riboflavin is recognized in that they are both active in enzyme formation after phosphorylation and combination with specific proteins. These enzymes are required for the proper oxidation and reduction processes of the body. Without these our most fundamental processes cannot proceed.

Folic acid and vitamin B_{12} are other vitamins of the Vitamin B Complex. They have been used in the treatment of various anemias and the latter in nutritional diseases of the nerves.

3. Viatmin C

Vitamin C is ascorbic acid; synonym: cevitamic acid. Source: fresh fruits and vegetables, especially lemons, oranges, grapefruit, tomatoes, strawberries, fresh—not pasteurized—cow's milk, because in the pasteurizing process most of the vitamin C is lost. The vitamin C content of cow's milk is much below that of human milk.

Lack of this vitamin causes scurvy and the principle of its application dates back to 1747, when James Lind, a British Navy surgeon, proved that orange and lemon juice prevented and cured this disease, formerly so common in long sea voyages. Seventy-five mg. of ascorbic acid is the recommended daily intake.

4. *Vitamin D*

Source: halibut- and cod-liver oil, and the short ultra-violet rays of the sun which convert 7-dehydrocholesterol of the skin into the active form which is then absorbed and is as effective as vitamin D fed and absorbed through the intestine. It is associated with the metabolism of calcium and phosphorus. Aside from the treatment of rickets it is claimed to reduce the susceptibility of the teeth to decay. Uses: vitamin D is specific in prevention as well as in the treatment of rickets, spasmophilia (infantile tetany) and osteomalacia (softening of the bone). Its lack may be concerned with fractures which are not uncommon in diabetics. It is valuable in pregnancy and lactation, and in fact vitamin requirements are doubled and quadrupled in these states and in growth, convalescence from long illnesses and especially in those who have been fed intravenously.

9

THE DIET OF DIABETIC INDIVIDUALS

THE diet in health is made up chiefly of carbohydrate; the diet in diabetes before the discovery of insulin necessarily was made up chiefly of fat. Insulin allows more carbohydrate, thus reducing dependence upon fat for calories which eaten in excess appear to lead to hardening of the arteries. It is just as important now as heretofore to avoid eating too much of any kind of food. *Diabetics should not be fat.* Diabetics should not grow thin suddenly, because that would mean they were living on a high fat—their own fat—diet.

A comparison of the components of a normal and a diabetic diet is given in Table 6.

TABLE 6.—NORMAL AND DIABETIC DIETS COMPARED. ADULT WEIGHING 132 POUNDS (60 KILOGRAMS) APPROXIMATELY 30 CALORIES PER KILOGRAM

Food	Comparison in grams		Comparison in calories	
	Normal	*Diabetic*	*Normal*	*Diabetic*
Carbohydrate.......	250	150*	1000	600
Protein............	60	75	240	300
Fat...............	60	90	540	810
Total............	370	315	1780	1710

*150 grams per day is the minimum carbohydrate allowance.

The normal individual weighing 60 kilograms, 132 pounds, takes 250 grams carbohydrate, and the average diabetic between 150 and 200 grams. Each takes from

50 to 100 grams of protein according to age. To make up for the slight loss of carbohydrate, the diabetic may increase the 60 grams of fat of the normal diet to 90 grams, often less and seldom more. Remembering that 1 gram of carbohydrate or protein yields 4 calories and

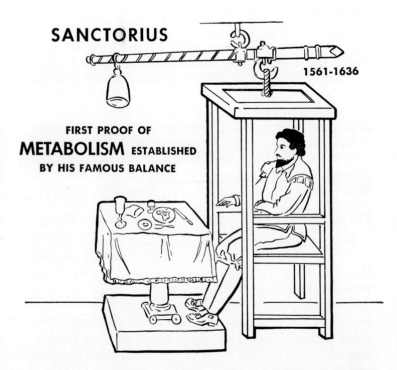

SANCTORIUS

1561-1636

FIRST PROOF OF
METABOLISM **ESTABLISHED**
BY HIS FAMOUS BALANCE

Fig. 13.—Sanctorius, 1561–1636, Sitting On His Steel-Yard Scales Found Less Was Given Off From The Body Than Was Taken In. This Inaugurated The Study Of Experimental Metabolism.

that 1 gram of fat yields 9 calories, one can arrive at the figures in the right half of Table 6. These diets are low rather than high, allow for no loss in preparation of food, and are for those with low or office activity.

7

Caloric Needs of the Diabetic

The diet of the diabetic patient should contain the minimum number of calories which the normal individual would require under similar conditions. Many normal individuals, in my opinion, actually live upon less than 30 calories per kilogram body weight, and repeatedly one sees diabetic patients over fifty years of age who live comfortably upon less for long periods. This is true only for the treated diabetic. If the patient is allowed more than the minimum amount of food there is far more likelihood that a portion will be lost, unassimilated, and appear as sugar in the urine. One of the first rules for the diabetic patient to learn is never to overeat. No matter whether upon a diet with low or high carbohydrate, low or high fat, all doctors agree that surplus food must be avoided. He should be a model in food conservation for his household.

The Estimation of the Carbohydrate in the Diabetic Diet

The quantity of carbohydrate in various foods is easily calculated and far more simply than is usually thought. (See Tables 3, 4 and 5, pages 65, 66 and 67, with accompanying text.)

A medium-sized orange, in which the pulp weighs 150 grams, or its equivalent is given most diabetics three times a day. An orange contains 10 per cent carbohydrate and thus the total in one orange is 15 grams and in 3 oranges 45 grams.

A slice of bread formerly weighed 30 grams (one ounce) but now often less and, depending upon the dryness of the bread, the carbohydrate varies from 50 per cent to 60 per cent and I suspect contains usually not far from 15 grams. If 3 slices, or 90 grams, are allowed we have 45 grams carbohydrate. Errors in reckoning carbohydrate readily occur if bread is not weighed.

Unless weighed, the slice is apt to grow larger rather than smaller.

A mixture of 3 per cent vegetables (four portions, approximately 600 grams, 20 ounces) accounts for about 20 grams more.

Cream 120 cc. ($\frac{1}{4}$ pint, 4 ounces) would contain 4 grams, and the same quantity of milk 6 grams carbohydrate.

Oatmeal, 1 large portion, 240 grams cooked, or 30 grams dry yields 20 grams carbohydrate. Other cereals weight for weight contain about one-fifth more carbohydrate. Altogether, we have carbohydrate in bread, 45, in fruits 45, in vegetables +20, in cream +4, in milk +6, in oatmeal +20, making a total of 140 grams, more or less. Fortunately, the content of carbohydrate in the 3 and 6 per cent groups of vegetables is so small that one is justified in the vast majority of cases in accepting an average figure of 20 grams for four large portions. It is true that there is considerable variation in the vegetables as classified in Table 3 but the average content in carbohydrate for all vegetables under one heading is not far from that represented, the error being in the assignment of too high rather than too low values. This does not hold for snap beans, because trouble often occurs from the snap beans containing the mature beans thus greatly increasing their content in carbohydrate. Many an unexplained trace of sugar in the urine has undoubtedly occurred in this way. In the same way squash, summer squash, and vegetable marrow vary in composition. Young vegetable marrow and young summer squash are safely included in the 3 per cent column, while any mature squash may be expected to run between 5 and 10 per cent. Be cautious also in the use of tomatoes.

One will not be very wrong if he considers the maximum amount of carbohydrate which a diabetic will secure from 3 per cent vegetables in the twenty-four hours as 20 grams. This is why in mild cases of diabetes it is unnecessary to weigh these vegetables, for it is improbable that a patient will eat too much of them. He is far more likely to eat too little. These vegetables are most desirable because of their content in vitamins, particularly vitamin C. One must never forget that a diabetic likes to eat and that he can seldom eat anything less harmful than 3 per cent vegetables. Tactful wives always provide their diabetic husbands not only with an abundance, but a wide variety of these vegetables and take infinite pains to get the best and to prepare them with the utmost care.

The Carbohydrate in Various Foods

1. THREE AND 6 PER CENT VEGETABLES.—These are of great value. (See Tables 3 and 5, pages 65 and 67.) Lettuce and cabbage are the most useful. By its bulk lettuce satisfies the appetite and the quantity allowed is unlimited. The introduction of iceberg lettuce was a great boon to diabetics. Cabbage is the poor man's 3 per cent vegetable. It can be eaten daily for months, raw and cooked. without repugnance. Case No. 866, in the pre-insulin era was sugar-free at the hospital with difficulty, but when he went to sea on a lumber schooner and lived almost exclusively on cabbage for his vegetable, he returned after one month not only with a sugar-free urine but with a normal blood sugar.

Artichokes are desirable. The French variety with the concentric leaves is to be classed as a 3 per cent vegetable; the Jerusalem artichokes which grow underground contain 16 per cent carbohydrate but this is partly as inulin—a precursor of levulose and so is well tolerated.

2. FRUIT.—Fruit is most desirable for a diabetic patient. The taste is agreeable, it serves instead of a dessert, and so relieves the patient of the embarrass-

ment of sitting idly at the table when others are eating. The best varieties of fruit for diabetic patients are grapefruit and strawberries, each containing about 7 per cent of carbohydrate, and oranges 10 per cent. These fruits are safer for the patient than apples (about 13 per cent), because they contain somewhat less carbohydrate and are more satisfying. Furthermore, it is less easy thoughtlessly to eat an orange than an apple. A small apple contains 1 tablespoonful of sugar and a large apple 3 tablespoonfuls. Before insulin was available I never had any success in allowing apples to diabetics and I taught all the children to reply to the question, "What should a diabetic do with an apple?" "Give it away." This is unnecessary today, but one must not forget an apple contains much sugar.

At present my patients use equivalents in their choice of fruits and certain other foods as representing 10 and 15 grams carbohydrate. (See Table 4, p. 66.) The values are approximate.

3. BREAD.—Insulin allows the diabetics bread. Previously few, save the old and mild diabetics, could take it without sugar appearing in the urine. Today practically all diabetics can have the equivalent of 1 slice at a meal. Bread is the staff of life, but it is often a broken reed for a diabetic. The easiest way dietetically to clear up sugar in the urine is temporarily to exclude all bread.

An error of 1 ounce in the weight of 3 per cent vegetables amounts to about 1 gram carbohydrate, and is negligible, but one slice of bread reaches from 12 to 18 grams, because slices of bread and the per cent of carbohydrate in each slice vary so much. If bread is toasted, it weighs less because it contains less water. The total carbohydrate in it remains the same although the per cent may rise to 60 or 70 per cent. If the bread is made without sugar and with water instead of milk, the carbohydrate content is lowered and may amount only to 45 per cent. Coarse breads if made without sweetening or milk would contain slightly less carbohydrate. Crackers and zwieback are even drier than toast, and in consequence the percentage of carbohydrate is nearer 70 per cent. This applies to Matsos of which one weighing 32 grams contains about the equivalent of a slice and a half of bread. The Jewish black bread contains about 45 per cent carbohydrate, but the slices of dark breads are often heavier than an ounce.

SUBSTITUTES FOR BREADS.—Many of the preparations of bread upon the market contain as great or even a greater quantity of carbohydrate than ordinary bread; a few contain less; but the percentage of carbohydrate may vary from time to time. Patients, and sometimes physicians, forget that substitutes for bread must be prescribed only in definite amounts. A "diabetic" bread should never be advised without a knowledge of its content of carbohydrate and protein.

BRAN BREADS.—Bran breads are so variable in content of carbohydrate because of added ingredients, so coarse and so liable to obstruct the bowels, that we no longer use them. Recently the carbohydrate in one bran muffin was estimated to be equal to 3 slices of white bread.

GLUTEN BREADS.—These breads are made by removing much of the starch from the flour. It is surprising how thoroughly this can be done. The large quantity of protein which all gluten breads contain is sometimes objectionable and always must be considered, if there is difficulty in making the urine of the patient sugar-free. Many gluten breads upon the market contain as much as 30 per cent carbohydrate but the protein may reach 40 per cent instead of 10 per cent in white bread. Thus in 30 grams or 1 slice there would be as much protein as in 2 eggs. As 58 per cent or more of protein can change to sugar the danger of the use of gluten breads is obvious. Bouchardat never wanted to be known as a "gluten bread doctor" although a hundred years ago he introduced it. He told his patients if in doubt about the carbohydrate in a food to test the urine an hour after eating it and thus learn whether it contained too much for them. English muffins and corn muffins are misleading because they weigh so much more than a slice of bread. They are more than half carbohydrate and therefore, should be weighed.

4. OATMEAL.—Oatmeal is two-thirds carbohydrate. In calculations one should be guided by the dry weight, because the different forms of oatmeal vary greatly in bulk and weight when cooked. It is a simple matter for a few days to weigh out 30 grams (1 ounce) of dry oatmeal, containing 20 grams carbohydrate, have it cooked and note the weight and bulk. Cooked oatmeal usually contains enough water to make the weight eight times that of the dry variety. A small saucerful, or half a cupful, of cooked oatmeal (weight 120 grams—4 ounces) contains the equivalent of dry oatmeal 15 grams ($\frac{1}{2}$ ounce) or 10 grams carbohydrate.

In weighing foods with the usual variety of scales one should never attempt to weigh out quantities as small as 5 grams. A more reliable result is obtained by weighing out multiples of 5 grams and then dividing into enough portions to make each portion 5 grams.

Whereas oatmeal, dry weight, is approximately two-thirds carbohydrate, most other cereals, especially those partially cooked and crisp and dry are three-quarters or more carbohydrate. Consequently in substituting another cereal for 30 grams oatmeal, lessen the amount to 25 grams.

5. MILK.—The carbohydrate in milk is in the form of lactose and can be reckoned at 5 per cent, or 1.5 grams per 30 cc., or 1 ounce. It is the same in skimmed milk, buttermilk and whey; but cream and koumiss contain about 3 per cent, or 1 gram carbohydrate to the ounce. Buttermilk and skimmed milk contain es-

sentially the same quantity of carbohydrate and protein as milk. (See page 90 and Table 26, page 288.)

6. POTATOES.—The variation in the percentage of carbohydrate in potatoes before and after cooking is negligible, save with potato chips, in which on account of the loss of water in their preparation the per cent of carbohydrate is more than doubled. In patoto chips the fat reaches nearly 40 per cent. Emphasis should be laid upon the comparatively small amount of carbohydrate (20 per cent) in potato in proportion to its bulk in comparison with the large percentage of carbohydrate in bread. Unfortunately it is not so easy to estimate carbohydrate in potatoes as in bread. A potato the size of an egg weighs about 60 grams and thus contains 12 grams carbohydrate. Many diabetic patients omit bread when they take potato. Boulin used potatoes far more than bread because of lower content of carbohydrate and so little protein.

7. NUTS.—Nuts containing 15 to 20 per cent carbohydrate are probably far less objectionable than most other foods with a similar carbohydrate content. This is due to the fact that in such nuts as almonds and peanuts a larger part of the carbohydrate is in the form of pentosan, galactan or other hemicelluloses, which probably do not readily form sugar. On the other hand, nuts are dangerous for a diabetic unless allowance is made for the considerable quantity of protein and the very large quantity of fat which they contain. Thirty grams (1 ounce) of castanas (Brazil nuts) represent about 6 nuts in which there are carbohydrate 2 grams, protein 5 grams, and *fat 20 grams, or 210 calories.* Ignorant diabetics often eat nuts as freely as they would 3 per cent vegetables and wonder why they gain weight, develop sugar in the urine and acid poisoning. Case No. 1930, quite mild when her treatment began, went home, ate nuts about as freely as some 3 per cent vegetables, and escaped diabetic coma, but only with

heroic treatment. Fifteen peanut kernels weigh about 30 grams and contain approximately carbohydrate 6 grams, protein 8 grams and fat 12 grams. They closely resemble American cheese 1 oz. plus 1 graham cracker or 2 saltines.

Protein in the Diabetic Diet

The quantity of protein required by diabetic patients varies with the age, weight and activity of the case as well as with the condition of the kidneys. It is a safe rule at the beginning of treatment to increase the protein gradually up to the same quantity as that required by a normal individual. This is approximately 1 to 1.5 grams per kilogram body weight for adults, but for children it may reach 3 grams.

Protein stimulates the metabolism more than any other kind of food, favors acidosis, and can lead to the formation of 58 or more grams of glucose for every 100 grams protein metabolized.

MEAT AND FISH.—These two articles constitute the chief sources of protein in the diabetic diet. The study of the chemical composition of these foods is simplified for the diabetic patient by the fact that carbohydrate is absent, except in liver and shell-fish. Even in liver the quantity of carbohydrate is almost negligible when we consider the amount and frequency with which this article of food is eaten. The analyses of liver and shell-fish will be found in Table 26.

The chief difficulty in computing the nutritive value of meat and fish is due to the varying content of fat. Thus, the edible portion of chicken may contain on the average 2.5 per cent of fat, whereas lean ham may contain 14 per cent of fat, fat ham as much as 50 per cent and smoked bacon 65 per cent, though lean smoked bacon 42 per cent. In general a mixture of cooked lean meats probably contains not far from 10 to 15 per cent of fat.

Fish differs from meat chiefly in the small quantity of fat. Even salmon, which contains more fat than most other fish, showed in its analysis only 12.8 per cent fat, shad 9.5 per cent, and herring and mackerel 7.1 per cent. In general, other kinds of fish show 6 per cent or less of fat. Halibut steak, for example, contains 5.2 per cent and cod 0.4 per cent. Preserved fish, however, is quite rich in fat; thus sardines contain 19.7 per cent. One egg and 30 grams of sardines are convenient equivalents.

The quantity of protein in meat also varies considerably and usually falls as the percentage of fat rises. A value of 20 per cent for protein in uncooked lean meat represents about the average, and this is increased when the meat is cooked. An ounce of cooked meat on the average contains about 7 grams of protein. The quantity of protein in fish is very slightly less than in meat.

Shell-fish make agreeable additions to the diet: (1) they are desirable because they are palatable; (2) they are bulky foods and so are satisfying; (3) they furnish a separate course at a meal. Half a dozen oysters or clams are quite sufficient. The edible portion of a medium-sized oyster on the shell weighs on the average $\frac{1}{2}$ ounce, and half a dozen oysters would amount to about 100 grams. The six would contain about 4 grams carbohydrate, 6 grams protein and 1 gram fat, the equivalent of 50 calories. Half a dozen clams on the shell (edible portion) weigh 35 grams and contain 0.7 gram carbohydrate, 3 grams protein and a negligible quantity of fat. The quantities of carbohydrate, protein and fat in oysters and clams are so negligible that usually one-half dozen, raw, can be disregarded.

Eggs.—Next to meat and fish, eggs are the most common source of protein for the diabetic. Reckon one egg as protein 6 grams and fat 6 grams. (See page 90).

CHEESE.—Cheese is a prolific source of protein and is to be recommended because of its lesser cost. Most varieties of cheese upon the market contain large percentages of fat. Even skimmed-milk cheese may contain as much as 15 per cent. The percentage of protein varies from 18.7 per cent in Neufchâtel cheese to 37.1 per cent in Dutch cheese, while the fat varies from 1 per cent in cottage cheese to 38.3 per cent in red American and to 38.9 per cent in Dutch cheese. Therefore, one must not be oblivious of the variety of cheese when eating an ounce of the same. In trying to lose weight be especially careful about the kind and amount of cheese in the diet. Disregard decimals generally when considering the components of foods. Values vary considerably.

BROTHS.—Broths are so extensively used for diabetic patients that their composition deserves notice. Jellylike broth contains a large quantity of protein in the form of gelatin, and when it was necessary, before the use of insulin, to reckon every gram of food a patient ate, its nutritive value could not be neglected. Gelatin is one of the least valuable of all the proteins. As a rule, the nutritive value of a broth can be disregarded. This will be the case if the broth is skimmed free of fat and obviously clear so as to be free from particles of meat fiber. Various canned bouillons and bouillon cubes contain very little nourishment, but make agreeable additions to the diet, and the sodium and potassium in them may be useful. (See page 112.)

Fat in the Diabetic Diet

Fat forms a large portion of the calories of the diabetic patient's diet, amounting to about half the total calories in the Basic Diet, Table 2, page 62, and to about a fourth or a third of the total calories even in those diets in which the carbohydrate is high and the fat correspondingly low. The discovery of insulin has lowered the fat in the diabetic's diet, because he can take more carbohydrate. Indirectly this is beneficial in that it lessens the danger of acidosis and diabetic coma and may retard the development of hardening of the arteries. It is possible that fat should be lowered to 30 per cent of the total calories, but as said before, there is not universal agreement. I think all will approve of using an unsaturated vegetable fat to replace some of the animal fat.

How much fat should a diabetic patient eat? This does not depend upon the capacity of the digestion. The safest answer would be: as little as possible above the normal quantity in order to maintain normal body weight.

Fat is most agreeably taken as cream, and cream which contains 20 per cent butter fat is usually easier to bear than a richer cream. The upper 120 cc. (4 ounces) of a quart bottle of milk which has stood for twenty-four hours is 20 per cent cream. Cream bought at the market as medium cream contains about 20 per cent butter fat, and heavy cream contains 38 per cent fat. It is seldom advisable to allow more than $\frac{1}{4}$ pint (120 cc.) of cream. One quarter pint of 20 per cent cream contains 24 grams of fat and the quantity of carbohydrate or of protein but little over 4 grams each and may be estimated in clinical work as 4 grams or 1 gram to the ounce. Oleo, butterine and nut margarine contain no sugar and have about the same percentage of fat as butter, and the cost is very much less. Lard is nearly 100 per cent fat. Crisco, also nearly 100 per cent fat, is often more welcome than lard, because of the lack of flavor. Oil is 100 per cent fat. Mineral oil is without nutritive value. Mineral oil can be used advantageously in place of olive oil in making salad dressings if one wishes to avoid the fat.

Mayonnaise Dressing

Yolk of egg....................	1
Mineral oil....................	1 cup
Juice of lemon.................	$\frac{1}{2}$
Salt, paprika, mustard, to taste	
Vinegar......................	1–2 tablespoonfuls

Beat yolk, add lemon juice, mustard, salt, paprika, then oil drop by drop until it is thoroughly worked in, not increasing amount until you are sure it will not separate. Add vinegar to proper consistency. Allow 2 dessertspoonfuls daily.

French Dressing

Mineral oil.............	$\frac{2}{3}$ cup	Salt
Vinegar...............	$\frac{1}{3}$ cup	Pepper
Saccharin.............	$\frac{1}{4}$ grain	Cayenne
Enough paprika to color.		

Mix in a small bottle which can be kept on the ice. Shake well before using.

Cod-liver oil is splendid for children and many children take 10 grams (2 teaspoonfuls) daily during the short days of winter. They thus obtain 90 calories and an abundance of vitamins A and D.

Danger of Fat to the Diabetic

Excess fat predisposes one to diabetes, makes treatment more difficult, formerly led to coma and death in two-thirds of the cases and now especially in unsaturated animal form contributes to disease of the arteries.

Advantages of a Weighed Diet

If a physician wishes to prescribe and a patient desires to live upon a definite diet, it is safer to weigh it than to guess at it. Freely granting that there are inaccuracies even in weighed diets, I believe they are most useful. Relatively from day to day a weighed diet will vary less than a guessed diet or grossly estimated diet. If one guesses at food values, one is apt to be careless in other ways and is tempted to overlook a specimen of urine when it contains a trace of sugar or even a greenish-yellow test. It is a comfort in the treatment of diabetes that one is dealing with facts and that results can be predicted. If sugar shows in the urine, there is a reason for it, and it is doing harm to the patient rather than good. In other words, the patient is getting worse instead of better.

I recommend to most diabetic patients at the commencement of their training to weigh their food. After a few days of weighing, they can select utensils which conform to the size of the portions of their own special diets and use them exclusively. By this means needless weighing is avoided. However, even then from time to time recourse to weighed diets will clear up inconsistencies in treatment in an obscure case.

Alcohol

Alcohol does not contain carbohydrate, but the oxidation of 1 gram in the body gives rise to 7 calories. If enough alcohol is taken by a diabetic to raise the diet above the caloric needs, sugar appears in the urine as it would after an excess of carbohydrate, protein or fat.

Theoretically alcohol might appear indicated in diabetes, but practically I believe patients do better without it. I notice that Bouchardat, that wonderful French diabetes clinician, as his experience grew, gave less and less alcohol. Furthermore, I think it far easier for a diabetic to exercise self-restraint without the use of alcohol than with it. It is certainly not needed in the diabetic dietary.

The pleasure which comes from the practice of medicine has increased materially since the restriction of the use of alcohol in the community and, despite allegations to the contrary, I believe the amount of alcohol consumed is less than forty years ago.

I base this upon my experience as a boy with the workmen in my father's factory in a country town, as a student in college and medical school, as a house officer in various hospitals, as a postgraduate medical student in Europe, as a physician attending medical gatherings and as a practitioner of medicine for sixty years. I believe modern machinery, the aeroplane, and the automobile will remove the alcoholic. When I read in a Boston paper (Nov. 1947) that 85 per cent of 1500 Boston children are being cared for by foster parents because alcohol disrupted their own homes, I am thankful that it is so exceptional for such a tragedy to occur with my patients. It is estimated that alcoholism costs Massachusetts $20,000,000 yearly and that the total cost is closer to $100,000,000.

A glass of beer contains about as much carbohydrate as the same quantity of milk and fully as much alcohol as a tablespoonful of whiskey. It lacks the protein and fat of milk. A glass of milk contains approximately 150 calories, but a glass of beer costs more and contains less.

There are few young men, much less young women or young doctors, who in looking for a job or a practice, or in seeking insurance, find it an asset to have it known that they drink. I do not want any such working for me.

Tobacco

I do not know of harm resulting from the use of tobacco save in the form of cigarettes. My impression is that they are harmful but I am not 100 per cent sure.

I think they contribute to complications in the eyes, arteries and kidneys. The most authoritative statement about cigarettes is contained in the following: "It is estimated that a man who smokes two packs of cigarettes a day has about one chance in ten of developing lung cancer, while a non-smoker has only one chance in 270 of having this disease. In addition to these ratios, the American Cancer Society's study also indicates that deaths from several other sites of cancer and from coronary heart disease were far higher among cigarette smokers than non-smokers. Among men in the American Cancer Society study, heavy cigarette smokers had about the same death rate as nonsmokers who were seven or eight years older. No one can predict what will happen to an individual but, in general, those who smoke less are those who live longer: To smoke or not to smoke is a personal decision."[1]

Liquids

It is rarely necessary to restrict the liquids in diabetes. The control of the diabetes, which diet, insulin, oral drugs and exercise provide, lessens the quantity of the sugar to be excreted and this usually leads to a corresponding diminution in thirst and in the volume of urine.

Sodium Chloride

Salt is of great service to the diabetic patient. If it is withdrawn from the diet the weight falls, due to excretion of water, and the skin and tissues of the patient become obviously dry. In the early days of the fasting treatment patients often lost much weight because water alone was allowed, and I learned of one case who lost 13 pounds in four days. Conversely, when

[1]American Cancer Society, Inc.: To smoke or not to snoke? New York, American Cancer Society, Inc., 521 West 57th. St., New York 19, N.Y.

salt-rich broths are freely given during fasting, it was not uncommon, particularly in the presence of acidosis, to see a patient gain weight, and invariably such patients feel better than those who lose.

The percentage of salt (sodium chloride) in the ocean and in the human blood is alike and the body tends to keep it constant. If the ingestion of salt is reduced then the volume of blood in the body is likewise reduced and the patient becomes dehydrated and loses weight. Conversely, if an extra quantity of salt is retained in the body the weight is increased, approximately one pound (one pint of water) for each teaspoonful of salt. In diabetic coma the tissues are very, very dry, and that is the reason why patients, if they suspect its approach, are advised to take a cup of broth, which contains a good deal of salt, hourly. So, too, in the treatment of coma, next to insulin, the injection of salt solution intravenously is of great importance. Prior and subsequent to operation, the same rules hold for liquids as for the non-diabetic. Often uncontrolled diabetes in an old man simulates disease of the prostate. Clear up the diabetes and the increased thirst and frequency of urination disappear. Rapid retention of water, thus overcoming the dehydration of untreated diabetes, may seriously impair vision by producing temporary shortsightedness (myopia). Consequently, do not purchase glasses when beginning treatment, but wait a month.

Polyuria, or excessive voiding of urine, persists in certain cases of diabetes. Usually a cause can be found in some peculiarity of diet such as an excess of salt. This happened with Case 1196 who continually voided large quantities of urine. Upon investigation it was found that he ingested 20 or more grams of salt, twice the ordinary quantity, bouillon cubes in variable numbers, and 21 half-grain saccharin tablets a day.

After operations the loss of water by the skin may

8

reach 2000 cc.—over two quarts—in twenty-four hours. The excretion by the lungs may amount to as much as 300 cc.—10 ounces.

From the above, it is evident that marked changes of weight can occur in a diabetic. As a matter of fact, these may be due simply to variations in the water content of the body, because it has been proved that the addition of one pound of actual tissue in a diabetic only takes place when some 1500 calories above ordinary needs are ingested.

During sleep a man loses about 30 grams, or an ounce an hour. In a football game a player with active exercise during an hour and fifteen minutes may lose as much as 6.4 kilograms, or 14 pounds.

The usual intake of salt is about 10 grams—10,000 milligrams. As the atomic weight of sodium is 23 and of chlorine 35, the quantity of sodium usually ingested and excreted would be about 4000 mg.

The first essential for a low sodium diet, which F. M. Allen showed so desirable in the treatment of high blood pressure, is to omit all salt either in the preparation of food or at the table. Especially avoid such foods as clear soups, bouillon cubes, canned soups, salad dressing, most sauces, molasses, olives and pickles, cheese, sour cream, ice cream and packaged puddings, kidneys, heart, brains, clams, crabmeat, lobster, shrimp and frozen fish.

Low sodium breads should be used exclusively, because a slice of ordinary bread contains 170 mg. of sodium. Even a cup (8 ounces) of milk contains 125 mg. but this can be replaced with Lonolac, which is sodium-free. One egg contains 40 mg. and is allowable, and one ounce of cooked meat contains 20 mg. sodium. Most vegetables, one-half cup containing 9 mg. sodium, are allowed, but beets, beet greens, celery, dandelion greens, kale, frozen peas, sauerkraut and spinach are excluded. Nearly all fresh fruits may be eaten, one serving containing only 2 mg. sodium, but raisins and figs must be omitted. Sweet butter, oils, lard are permitted, and for seasoning caraway, cinnamon, lemon juice, dry mustard, nutmeg, paprika, parsley, pepper, pimiento, saccharin, sage, thyme, vanilla extract and vinegar. Substitutes for salt are Diasal and Cosalt.

Two detailed diets follow, one low in sodium, 1–2 grams (1000–2000 mg.), and the other a minimal sodium diet containing 200 mg. (See Tables 7 and 8, pp. 116, 117.)

Potassium

Potassium is essential to life. It is remarkable that without a thought on our part the proper balance of its intake and outgo is maintained. In general, it is only when disease or man interferes and profoundly manipulates the diet that disturbances result. If the normal level of potassium—3.1 to 4.5 mEq. per liter—in the blood serum is increased or decreased, serious disturbances occur. The normal amount of potassium ingested daily is about 3 to 4 grams, or about that of sodium. Ten to 20 per cent of the potassium is lost in the feces, or rather more than the nitrogen of the diet.

Potassium is distinctively a substance which is contained in the cells unlike sodium which is extracellular. Potassium accompanies glucose as the latter is deposited as glycogen in tissues. Death can occur from a low or a high serum potassium. The low potassium in the serum may result when it is depleted due to lack of its ingestion following surgical operations, prolonged vomiting, diarrhea or through prolonged drainage of the alimentary tract. A dangerously low value for potassium in diabetic coma occurs only when the coma is prolonged and glucose is administered in the course of treatment. Glucose carries potassium with it into the cell.

TABLE 7.—LOW SODIUM DIET (1–2 GRAMS NA)

This diet contains approximately 200 grams of carbohydrate, 70 grams of protein, 100 grams of fat, and 2000 calories. All food is prepared and served without salt.

Type of Food	Foods Allowed	Foods Avoided
Beverage	Any beverage; limit milk to one pint daily including that used in cooking	Milk in excess of one pint
Bread	Salt-free bread and crackers	Bread or crackers made with baking powder, baking soda, or salt
Cereals	Salt-free cooked cereal, puffed rice, puffed wheat, shredded wheat	Any other
Desserts	Salt-free desserts; custards and ice cream made from milk allowance; unsalted fruit pies; puddings, rennet desserts	Desserts prepared with salt, baking powder, baking soda, or egg whites
Fat	Salt-free butter; cream; lard; oil; salt-free salad dressing, vegetable fat	Salted butter; bacon fat; salted salad dressing
Fruit	Any juice; canned, cooked or raw fruit	None
Meat, egg or cheese	Any meat, liver, poultry or fresh fish that is not smoked or prepared with salt	Salted meats, ham; bacon; shellfish except oysters; glandular meat except liver; smoked or canned meats or fish; all cheese
Potato or Substitute	Potato; hominy; macaroni; noodles, rice; spaghetti, all prepared without salt	Fried potato; potato chips
Soup	Salt-free broth or cream soups made from milk allowance	Soup made with salt
Sweet	Candy; jam and jelly, sugar; syrup	None
Vegetable	Any raw, frozen or cooked vegetable or juice prepared without salt; any vegetable or juice canned without salt	Vegetables prepared or canned with salt
Miscellaneous	Cocoa; unsalted cream sauce; herbs; spices; vinegar; unsalted nuts	Catsup; chili sauce; mustard; olives, peanut butter, pickles; popcorn; relishes; salt

I am indebted to Miss Effie May Winger, Chief Dietician, New England Deaconess Hospital, for the Low and Minimal Sodium Diets.

TABLE 8.—MINIMAL SODIUM DIET (200 MILLIGRAMS)

This diet contains approximately 225 grams of carbohydrate, 70 grams of protein, 90 grams of fat, and 2000 calories. All food is prepared and served without salt in the amounts allowed. If whole milk is substituted for Lonolac, the sodium content of this diet will be increased to approximately 450 milligrams.

Type of Food	Foods Allowed	Foods Avoided
Beverage	Carbonated beverage; cereal beverage; coffee; tea; Lonolac	Milk; milk drinks
Bread	Salt-free bread and crackers	Bread or crackers made with baking powder, baking soda, eggs or salt
Cereal	Salt-free cooked Ralston, Maltex, Pettyjohn, Wheatena, cornmeal, oatmeal, puffed wheat, puffed rice, shredded wheat	All others
Dessert	Gelatin desserts made from plain gelatin; unsalted pie from fruit allowed; fruit tapioca pudding	Desserts made with egg, milk, baking powder, or baking soda; prepared gelatin desserts
Fat	Salt-free butter; salt-free salad dressing without egg white	Any other
Fruit	Any fruit juice canned, cooked or raw fruit	None
Meat, Egg or Cheese	Beef; chicken, lamb, liver, pork, veal, fresh fish, oysters, turkey, 4 oz. daily prepared without salt; egg, not more than 1 daily in place of 1 oz. meat	Salted meat; smoked or canned meats or fish; shellfish except oysters; glandular meat except liver; eggs except as allowed; all cheese
Potato or Substitute	Potato, macaroni, noddles, rice, spaghetti; all prepared without salt	Fried potato; potato chips; hominy
Soup	Unsalted soup made from vegetables allowed	All other
Sweet	Candy; honey; jam or jelly; sugar	Molasses; syrup
Vegetable	Most fresh and frozen vegetables prepared without salt	Beets and beet greens, celery, chard, dandelion greens, spinach, white turnip and turnip greens in all forms; frozen peas, any vegetable canned with salt

Calcium (Lime)

Acidosis if prolonged depletes the stores of alkali in the body and this process extends even to the bones. This in itself would not be harmful if the diet replenished the calcium and magnesium so lost, but in this respect it may fail, because milk, the great source of calcium, is so often restricted in treatment. Such deprivation may result in the decalcification of the bones to such a degree that a slight trauma may lead to a fracture. If such a fracture occurs in the spine of an elderly, feeble patient, the resulting pain may be so slight at the time that it will be unnoticed and later can be looked back upon as a spontaneous fracture. The incidence of fractures in our cases of diabetes is considerable, although possibly not greater than among non-diabetic persons of comparable ages. The National Research Council recommends 1 gram calcium in the diet daily. An ordinary hospital diet without milk and eggs or their products contains about 0.4 gram calcium, but milk 90 cc., cream 120 cc., American cheese 10 grams, or 3 eggs each contain 0.1 gram. so that it is easy to bring the calcium up to a proper figure. Pregnant and nursing women require nearly twice as much calcium and that is why their diet must contain more milk.

Phosphorus

If the calcium is adequate in the diet, so far as I am aware one need not prescribe phosphorus.

Iron

In diabetics today anemia is noted with about the same frequency as in non-diabetics. Iron is especially abundant in liver, meat, navy beans, lima beans, eggs, beef, prunes, whole wheat. Unfortunately, molasses, which is rich in iron, finds no place in the diabetic diet.

Pregnant mothers need iron and, in fact, women require more iron than do men and pregnant women twice as much as non-pregnant women.

DIETETIC SUGGESTIONS, RECIPES AND MENUS

The modern diabetic has little need for diabetic recipes, because the diabetic diet today is sufficiently varied and liberal to be both palatable and satisfying. Plain foods well cooked are enjoyed the most, and the taste for such grows rather than wanes. It is both less conspicuous and less troublesome to select the food from the diet served the rest of the family and with intelligence this can be done. The less a diabetic alters the essentials of the standard diet the easier it is for him in the long run to adhere to it.

Desserts

Desserts can often be made with gelatin and this may be flavored with coffee, lemon, rhubarb, or cracked cocoa. D-Zerta is useful. Jello may contain sugar. Look out! In preparing gelatin desserts if saccharin is used it should be added as late as possible during the cooking for it is apt to become bitter with heat. It is always a safe rule to add too little rather than too much saccharin. Sucaryl is preferred by many.

Lunches

In planning meals or lunches, one can always refer to Tables 3, 4, 5 and 26 for details. Reckoning is easy when one remembers that bread 1 slice contains about carbohydrate 15 grams and protein 2.5 grams, a medium-sized orange carbohydrate 15 grams, vegetables in the 3 per cent and 6 per cent groups 4 liberal portions about carbohydrate 20 and protein 6 grams, milk 1 glass (8 oz., 240 cc.) carbohydrate 12, protein 8, fat 8 grams, one egg protein 6 and fat 6 grams, and meat, fish or cheese approximately protein 7 and fat 5 grams to each ounce (30 grams), butter fat 25 grams in each ounce, or 5 grams in a small serving.

Extracts

In making agar jelly, gelatin and other desserts, flavoring extracts can be used, I teaspoonful to 1 pint.

Sea moss farina and Irish moss are usually allowable for diabetic patients. Most of the carbohydrate in these materials is quite inert in the body. Unfortunately these products are sometimes adulterated.

Seasoning

The proper seasoning of the food helps the diabetic patient. Horseradish, to be sure, contains 10 per cent carbohydrate, but it would take at least 2 teaspoonfuls to contain a gram, and probaby far more. Sour pickles are allowable, and other pickles made from the group of 3 per cent vegetables, provided one is assured that they have been prepared without sweetening. Mint, capers, curry, tarragon vinegar, distilled vinegar, bay leaf, cloves, ginger, mustard, paprika, anise seed, caraway seed, celery salt and onion extract may all be used as seasoning.

There are many preserved and canned foods on the market for diabetics. Be sure to note the exact composition on the label.

Recipes for diabetics are constantly appearing in the publications of diabetic lay societies and in the data distributed by the manufacturers of insulin. These are available for the asking.

10

THE TREATMENT OF DIABETES

DIET—INSULIN—BLOOD-SUGAR-LOWERING DRUGS—EXERCISE

Who learns and learns,
Yet does not what he knows,
Is one who plows and plows
Yet never sows.[1]

I LOOK upon the diabetic as a charioteer and his chariot as drawn by three steeds named (1) Diet, (2) Insulin and (3) Exercise. It takes skill to drive one horse, intelligence to manage a team of two, but a man must be a very good teamster who can get all three to pull together and to succeed he needs instruction and practice. (See Figs. 36, 37 and 38 on pages 253, 254.) Indeed in this year 1959 there is another spare horse, an oral blood-sugar-lowering drug, but just how much of the load it will pull time alone can tell. (See page 150.)

To get rid of the symptoms of diabetes—weakness, loss of weight, thirst, hunger, local irritation, frequency of urination—one must prevent the loss of sugar in the urine. If this can be done by a diet moderately restricted in sugar and starch and limited in quantity, well and good, but if not, it is better to take insulin or oral drugs. By reducing the carbohydrate in the diet to a slice of bread and an orange at a meal with liberal quantities of vegetables in the 3 per cent carbohydrate group and $\frac{1}{2}$ cup of milk at a meal plus a reasonable allowance for meat, eggs, fish, cheese and butter, this

[1] Translated from the Persian by James Phinney Baxter.

can often be accomplished provided the patient adheres to it for several days. If such a diet should be increased by a half portion of cereal and a small potato it would be a safe diet for the average diabetic for a lifetime. A very mild diabetic could take half again as much carbohydrate and it would be extraordinary for any diabetic to need twice as much. The first diet mentioned would contain carbohydrate 120–130 grams, the second 150–165 grams and the third 225 grams. These diets are described on pages 62–67, Tables 2 and 5, both in weights as well as in portions.

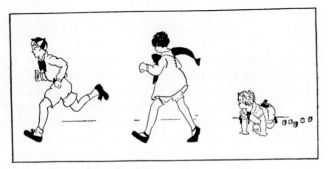

Fig. 14.—Sugar enters the blood as fast as a child runs.
  Starch enters the blood as fast as a child walks.
  The starch in vegetables enters the blood as slowly as a child creeps.

If a patient is fat and forty, persistence in a diet low in carbohydrate as well as calories will usually render him sugar-free and free from symptoms, but this might take several weeks and the loss of many pounds of weight. Such a diet would not be helpful to the underweight, to young people or to children. For all these latter groups it is desirable to give insulin or oral drugs at the start and even to most of the others at least temporarily in order to enable them to regain health and strength quickly. But just because one can secure such results comfortably and rapidly for the patient with diet and insulin, it should not be forgotten that restricting the diet alone can accomplish much.

The third factor in treatment—exercise—gains in importance as the disease begins to come under control.

What I learned before we had insulin, in those dire days of treatment by fasting and undernutrition of diabetics, serves me in good stead still. Some of these simple facts I will record at once.

Eat Less Sugar and Starch

Sugar in the urine comes chiefly from sugar and starch in the food. Therefore, most diabetics must take less sugar and starch (carbohydrate) at their meals than normal individuals. Sugar and starch act almost alike in the body because the starch of the food changes to sugar soon after it is eaten. If the food is composed of cooked starch, the change goes on very rapidly. Cereals, rice, macaroni, breads and potato contain so high a percentage of starch that they change quickly to sugar in the digestive tract, whereas the coarser vegetables contain so little starch and this is so closely mixed with the fiber of the vegetables that its transformation goes on much more gradually. A lump of sugar might be said, figuratively, to *run* into the blood; a tablespoonful of cooked oatmeal, which contains the same amount of sugar as the lump, to *walk* into the blood; the starch in a large dish of lettuce or cabbage, which is also equivalent to the lump of sugar or to the tablespoonful of oatmeal—would be transformed to sugar so slowly in the course of digestion that it would *creep* into the blood. This is very important, because it explains why diabetics should abhor sugar, measure carefully any bread, cereal, potato, rice or macaroni, but eat 3 per cent vegetables freely. One should select those foods which will not suddenly overload the blood with sugar, because thus there is less chance for it to escape through the kidneys into the urine. Similarly, spread the meals far apart and thus also avoid much carbohydrate at any time. Take an early breakfast and a late evening meal. Houssay has shown that rats made susceptible to diabetes by alloxan were more likely to develop it if all the food was given at one meal instead of distributed through the entire twenty-four hours.

Eat More Vegetables

The safest vegetables, because they contain the least carbohydrate, are lettuce, cucumbers, spinach and asparagus. Others follow in order of percentage of carbohydrate such as celery, tomatoes, cabbage and young snap beans. These vegetables belong to the group of 3 per cent vagetables. Then come the 6 per cent vegetables—pumpkin, turnip, squash, beets, carrots, onions, very young green peas. The 15 per cent vegetables are mature peas, Jerusalem artichokes, parsnips, lima beans. Vegetables which contain 20 per cent of carbohydrate are potatoes, shell beans, corn. (See Table 3.) The 20 per cent vegetables must be used cautiously and the results of their use learned by tests of the urine one to two hours after a meal.

The 3 per cent vegetables are a comfort to a diabetic, because they contain so little carbohydrate that they can be eaten freely; they are satisfying because of their bulk, and they are rich in vitamins A, B, and C. For practical purposes the quantity is unlimited.

Test the Effect of Change in Diet by Examination of Urine for Sugar

If the change in diet makes the urine free from sugar (sugar-free) and body weight and strength are satisfactory, the patient is doing well. If the carbohydrate in a meal is too great, sugar will show in the urine in one hour. To know whether the urine is sugar-free the patient should learn to test the urine for sugar. This is easily done and the method is described on pages 275–276. If sugar is found in the urine voided after one meal, but not after the others, the carbohydrate can be lowered at that one meal and raised at the others.

Do Not Lower Carbohydrate Too Much

Reduction in carbohydrate must not be too great, because either too much weight will be lost or, if the carbohydrate is replaced by extra protein and fat to prevent this, danger can result from acid posioning, because then one forces the body to depend too much upon fat. Fifty years ago I advised patients to reduce the carbohydrate greatly to become sugar-free and gave them much fat to make up for it; later I reduced carbohydrates less, because Dr. F. M. Allen proved it was not necessary to reduce the carbohydrate so much if the total diet was restricted. As a result often a diabetic could take one-third, one-half and often two-thirds of the carbohydrate which would be proper in health. It is still possible to drive the sugar out of the urine of most patients by prescribing very little carbohydrate, but I believe the patient is better off if he does not lower it below 150 grams, even if he must take insulin to get the benefit of it. For this reason patients must learn not only what kinds of food to eat, but also how much, and the more they know, the easier it is for them to live with safety and comfort.

It is not very difficult to learn what kind and how much of the different varieties of food one should take. The carbohydrate is reduced one-half of that taken in health. The protein (meat, fish, eggs, cheese) would be the same or a little more or less than the individual ordinarily eats. The fat would be increased sufficiently to enable the patient to maintain the proper weight.

Yet it is not all quite so simple. The diet must be planned so that there will be few exceptions to the rule that the urine must be free from sugar. If necessary to accomplish this, rather than reduce the carbohydrate below 150 grams I think it wiser for the patient to take advantage of the discovery of insulin or oral drugs. The rule for a sugar-free urine may be modified at times for a few hours in the day for those away from home and in active work to prevent a low blood sugar, but I dislike to see more than a green or greenish-yellow test with Benedict's solution or more than a few grams (5 or 10 per cent) of the total carbohydrate in the diet so lost; more than that usually implies inadequate or poor treatment. Writing in 1959, my aim, more than ever is to keep the urine sugar-free and blood sugar normal in order to prevent complications later on.

Division of Carbohydrate Between the Three Meals

The division of the carbohydrate between the three meals is important. The least amount, perhaps one-fifth of the total for the day, should be given at breakfast, leaving two-fifths for each of the other two meals, with allowances from these for small quantities of food between meals and at bedtime.

Diabetes is Most Severe Early in the Morning

It is then that the patient shows sugar in the urine after less food than at any other time of the day. In the morning before breakfast he has very little glycogen (animal starch) stored in the liver, and that is always bad for a diabetic. There are two reasons for this. First, during the night the body has been without carbo-hydrate food from which glycogen is most readily made, and although a certain quantity can be obtained from the breakdown of protein, one does not wish to force the destruction of body tissue to produce this. Second, the body has little insulin, either its own or that artificially administered early in the morning unless protamine zinc insulin is employed, because the quick insulins, regular and crystalline, and even the intermediate insulins, Globin, Lente and NPH, do not act as powerfully through the latter hours of the night. Protamine zinc insulin is a sheet anchor to a diabetic because it exerts an effect for nearly two days and therefore the diabetes is always to some extent controlled.

Glycogen, animal starch, in the liver of a diabetic is like gold in the bank for a business man. Insulin helps to deposit it. Without capital in the form of glycogen in the liver a diabetic is as badly off as a business man without gold. One can carry the analogy still further. A diabetic without glycogen is as ill-fitted to meet diabetic coma as a business man without gold is to meet a business crisis. Therefore, never try to do a big business in carbohydrate at that time of the day when your glycogen capital is small.

Theoretically the form in which the patient takes his carbohydrate makes no difference, but it makes a great deal of difference practically. Already we have commented upon the rapidity with which pure sugar leaves the stomach and enters the blood and the more gradual passage of starch in the form of bread and potatoes and the slowness in which the carbohydrate in vegetables is absorbed. But there is another reason. The diabetic is human when he eats. Oatmeal although it contains much carbohydrate is served but once a day and a patient is not so easily tempted to break his diet with it as with bread. Out of sight out of mind. The same holds true of grapefruit as compared with apples. Boys and men, as mothers and wives know, love to eat. Therefore give them food which takes time to consume —such as raw fruits instead of juices, and coarse vegetables instead of potatoes.

The development of the full power of the patient to

utilize carbohydrate is favored by diets somewhat low in protein and fat. Often one is gratified to see the patients do far better than was at first anticipated. Overeating of any kind of food lowers the power of the diabetic to assimilate carbohydrate. This is one of Allen's great contributions. Elderly diabetics may be allowably discharged after a brief hospital stay without the urine becoming quite sugar-free or the blood sugar absolutely normal. This is done with the expectation, which experience has justified, that persistence in a diet of slight undernutrition will lead to the disappearance of the slight quantity of sugar in the urine. Time accomplishes what heroic treatment often fails to secure. In reality these patients demonstrate the recuperative power of the insulin-secreting cells of the pancreas, such as one observes after the abatement of an infection or of an injudicious diet which has needlessly brought acid poisoning and made the diabetes worse.

The Recuperative Power of the Pancreas

Years ago we seldom thought this possible, although Naunyn had observed it. He wrote that occasionally the case which appears severe, if aggressively treated may later surprise one by becoming mild. But the mild case neglected always gets severe. Brush in 1944 pointed out that even children, near the onset of their diabetes, if enough insulin was given so that their own pancreas did not need to produce any and thus was rested, they would regain their power to take carbohydrate and often need no insulin at all. Later, in a few months this remission would disappear. Today, there are many other proofs that the pancreas can recuperate if rested. Therefore, with all new cases of diabetes and even old cases, one looks for a remission and overtreats rather than undertreats the diabetes. I believe we are near the day when we can hope to advance the treatment of diabetes more than we have hitherto known how to do.

Professor Boulin wrote, don't consider diabetes always irreversible. Stop saying: "Le médecin arrive trop tard." (The doctor arrives too late.)

Standard Diabetic Diets

To save time for doctors and nurses certain standard diets are frequently used at the New England Deaconess Hospital. Several of these are shown on pages 62, 66, 126. The patient receives a portion of fruit and bread or cereal at each of his three meals. In addition an egg and sometimes bacon for breakfast; at noon and night meat or fish and 3 and 6 per cent vegetables, and during the day a limited quantity of butter, cream, milk and perhaps potato. Often less is desired at breakfast and one-half of the oatmeal or one-half of the bread can be omitted and used for a mid-morning lunch. Similarly, a little carbohydrate can be saved out for an afternoon tea and retiring lunch. If grapefruit or strawberries, instead of an orange, are used for breakfast, one gains 5 grams of carbohydrate for later in the day.

The meals of a diabetic should be far apart with lunches in the mid-morning, mid-afternoon and upon retiring. By this means the diet is better tolerated, appetite satisfied and one avoids the annoyance of an insulin reaction. In a hospital a diabetic is greatly handicapped if his breakfast is served at 8:00 A.M. and his supper at 5 P.M. An early breakfast and a late evening meal are desirable for a diabetic. Children do not forget the advantage of a late supper.

Fasting is a very efficient way in which to banish the sugar from the urine, but I do not like to use it. During fasting the patient is almost devoid of carbohydrate, because there is so little stored in the body of a diabetic. Actually he is living almost wholly upon his own body

9

fat. He is thus on a very low-carbohydrate but very high-fat diet and nearly all agree that is bad for him.

Should it be desired to give a diet low in fat and high in carbohydrate, cream, bacon and cheese are omitted and butter reduced to 15 grams or none. Naturally fat meats, fat fish and oil would be debarred. The carbohydrate could be increased by the addition of bread or substitutes for it. Sometimes I think it is forgotten that every person in the world began life and continued it for many months upon a diet which contained relatively large proportions of protein and fat to carbohydrate. Thus, the composition of 1 quart, actually 1 liter (1000 cc.), of human milk is approximately carbohydrate 70 grams, protein 15 grams, and fat 40 grams, and of cow's milk carbohydrate 50 grams, protein 35 grams, and fat 35 grams. I can't believe we should lower the fat under 40 grams.

INSULIN: USES AND ABUSES

Treatment with Insulin

WHO SHOULD USE IT.—If a diabetic is not happy, energetic and a joy to himself and to his family, and his urine sugar-free, he had better take insulin. The chances are overwhelming that it will do him good. Even if he does not actually require it or only needs it temporarily, it is a good plan to learn how to use it, because then he will be ready for emergencies, such as infections and operations which later he may have to face. Insulin allows a diabetic to eat more, to work more, to sleep undisturbed, to ward off complications of diabetes, to postpone the coming on of old age and by living long, either largely to outlive the symptoms of diabetes and perhaps to give up insulin or at least to approach more nearly to that Golden Age when diabetes will be more easily treated or perhaps cured.

I wrote the preceding paragraph years ago and it holds true in 1959, but I can add to it. I am convinced that a diabetic whose disease is controlled with carbohydrate 150 grams or more in his diet, plus insulin, is less likely to grow old prematurely than when controlled with carbohydrate 100 grams and no insulin. As for the Golden Age, I cannot say protamine zinc insulin, NPH, Lente and Globin insulins brought it, but they certainly have made it less remote. It will pay any diabetic to keep alive, and to follow treatment carefully so as to profit by new discoveries which are sure to come. See Chapter 2 for a description of 85 Quarter Century Victory Medal cases who were free from complications after 25 years, and Chapter 3 for the use of the oral drugs.

Insulin, the second horse of the diabetic's chariot, is a clever steed, practically never fails to do what is asked, but unless understood, may run away with the driver. One needs a good many lessons and much practice to ride a prancing horse, and this Insulin horse is no exception. Just as there are different kinds of horses, so there are different types of insulin. The race-horse variety of insulin is the quick-acting regular or crystalline insulin, while the draft-horse is matched by the slow-acting protamine zinc insulin. Intermediate insulins, Globin, Lente and NPH, come in between.

At the present writing the insulin treatment of new cases of diabetes can begin with 8 units of NPH insulin, which is increased at least 4 to 12 units every day or every other day until the urine is sugar-free on rising. If the percentage of sugar in the urine or blood is high, one may begin with 30 or even more units and even supplement it with crystalline insulin, bearing in mind the dangers of an approaching coma or insulin reaction. If one proceeds slowly, there is a better chance to observe what the change in diet is accomplishing.

Regular Insulin

Regular insulin, the first insulin manufactured, acts rapidly, is most powerful one hour after injection, but its effect wears off in about six hours. Crystalline insulin, sold as "solution of zinc insulin crystals," is like it, acts fully as promptly and persists for an hour or so longer. Crystalline and regular insulins are "quick- and short-acting" insulins in contrast to the "slow- and long-acting" protamine zinc insulin which is so valuable in

TABLE 9.—ACTION OF VARIOUS INSULINS.

Regular, Crystalline, Protamine Zinc, Globin,
Lente and NPH Insulins

Type of Insulin	Year Marketed	Greatest Intensity of Action in Hours	Duration of Action in Hours
Regular...............	1922	1–2	6
Crystalline............	1936	1–2	7
Protamine Zinc.........	1936	12	26–48
Globin...............	1939	8–10	18–24
NPH.................	1950	8–10	26–30
Lente................	1954	8–10	26–30
Semilente.............	1954	slow	12–18
Ultralente.............	1954	Very slow	36 plus

treatment, because one injection of this twenty-four-hour acting insulin will replace two or three injections of the short-acting. The protamine zinc insulin slowly and gradually shows its power to lower the blood sugar in the first six hours, but continues to do so for nearly forty-eight hours. To control a severe case of diabetes would require three or four doses of quick insulin, and quick insulin would be the insulin to use to bring a patient out of diabetic coma. On the other hand, the slow protamine zinc insulin (PZI) is the insulin for many patients because it exerts a control of the diabetes for the entire day. It may not be strong enough to offset all the carbohydrate food taken at the three meals. In that event and in any case it is a good plan to reduce the carbohydrate at meals and prescribe a very light lunch in the forenoon, late afternoon, and upon retiring. If this does not suffice to keep the urine sugar-free, then the indication is to add a few units of quick insulin before breakfast.

Period of Action of Regular and Crystalline Insulin

Since regular or crystalline insulin acts most power-fully about one hour after it is injected, it is given one-half hour before a meal in order to meet the high tide of sugar in the blood which occurs at one-half hour after a meal. In this way its greatest effect is exerted when the products of the meal are collected in the blood. Insulin's task is to keep the blood sugar between 0.10 (100 mg.) per cent and 0.15 (150 mg.) per cent.

NPH[1] Insulin, Globin and Lente Insulin

These insulins are intermediate in action between the quick-acting regular and crystalline insulins on the one hand and the slow-acting protamine zinc insulin on the other. Their most marked effect is about eight hours after injection, and so if given before breakfast the lowest blood sugar will be found in the mid- or late after-noon. This is the time of the day in which one must especially guard against reactions with these insulins. The duration of action of Globin insulin is a little less than twenty-four hours and NPH and Lente insulin a little over twenty-four hours. Doctors, therefore, often find moderately severe cases can be controlled with these intermediate insulins, although the possibility

[1] NPH signifies Neutral Protamine Hagedorn Insulin.

always exists of a reaction in the afternoon or, because of their shorter duration, an elevated blood sugar before breakfast.

If the intermediate insulins are ineffective, regular or crystalline insulin can be given in small quantity by *separate* injection with the protamine zinc insulin before breakfast, or by directly combining it with NPH or Globin insulin. Both regular and crystalline insulins lose their identity when mixed with protamine zinc insulin, because they unite with its surplus protamine, but they retain their individual character if added to NPH, Globin, or Lente insulin.

If a diabetic taking regular insulin divided his carbohydrate between three meals as follows, 30–60–60 grams, he should change with protamine zinc insulin to three meals and three lunches, perhaps as follows, 30–(10)-45–(10)–45–(10) in which the grams in parentheses represent lunches in the forenoon, afternoon and evening. By an arrangement somewhat similar to the above the carbohydrate of the meals could be spread out over a still longer period. It is indeed advantageous for a diabetic taking PZI to have his meals far apart—an early breakfast and a late evening meal. If sugar still appears in the urine, despite dietetic rearrangement, then, as said above, one would give the quick crystalline insulin before breakfast at the same time as the protamine zinc and in that way control the disease. Until the discovery of protamine zinc insulin, most patients took insulin two or three times daily and occasionally four times. Rarely a dose would be necessary even during the night, and 4 A.M. was not so unusual an hour especially for children. It was quite common for patients to take 2 to 8 units upon retiring, but even then the blood sugar might fail to be normal on waking in the morning. Protamine zinc insulin, given before breakfast, corrects these inconveniences because it acts all the time—"works while you sleep"—and with it the blood sugar should be normal before breakfast

Period of Action of Protamine Zinc Insulin

Protamine zinc insulin, unlike regular insulin, acts a long time—for twenty-four hours or more, at times even forty-eight hours—and therefore is required but once a day. It is conceivable an insulin can be prepared which will last much longer. Certainly we can be sure that progress in the preparation of insulin has not ceased. Patients who have never taken insulin readily learn to get the full benefit of it. They usually begin with 8 units before breakfast and then increase daily or every few days by 4 or 8 units up to even 32 units if necessary. If the diabetes is still uncontrolled, it is usually wiser to shift to NPH insulin which acts slightly more rapidly, and if this does not prove satisfactory, to add RI or CI insulin to the NPH. If RI or CI is added to PZI, one must allow for about half of it being changed to PZI, thus leaving only half of the added dose serving as a quick-acting insulin.

Protamine zinc insulin exerts its power so slowly and so slightly at one time that its good effects are not seen for three or more days after it has been begun. The first day's dose overlaps in action that of the second day and even reaches the third, so that one should not be discouraged if one must wait several days for results. It does not cumulate in the body.

Diabetics, save those most mild, have less capacity to utilize food at breakfast. This is due to the blood sugar rising during the night. Quick insulin before the evening meal would not correct this and even if taken at retiring would have lost its effect before morning. Protamine zinc insulin in such a case would bring the blood to normal before breakfast, because it would act all night. One decides about the dose of protamine zinc insulin by the presence or absence of sugar in the urine on rising or, better, by a specimen voided one-half hour later

If a patient taking protamine zinc insulin has any of the signs of a reaction, such as headache, nausea, weakness or drowsiness upon waking in the morning, it is a good plan for him to take the fruit, usually eaten at breakfast, at once upon awakening and at the same time the insulin is injected. The low blood sugar also may be avoided by increasing the lunch on retiring or by lowering the amount of insulin.

ADDITIONAL COMMENTS ON THE USE OF INSULIN

Insulin will keep unless frozen or overheated, but it is wiser to place all of it in the refrigerator save the actual vial in daily use.

The dosage of insulin of any kind is variable. Patients and doctors must remember that insulin always works. (Perhaps one case in a thousand is temporarily almost totally resistant.) Some patients need very little, others a great deal, and the insulin requirement of the same individual may vary from hour to hour and day to day. It is a wonder how uniformly it acts. The dose is prescribed to get the result required and fortunately this can be determined by examination of the urine and blood. There is no hard and fast rule for dosage. One must test each patient individually, remembering that the dose determined upon one day may later require reduction or, if a complication arises, an increase. This is one of the reasons why patients should understand the treatment of diabetes.

Small doses of insulin do the most good per unit. For example, the first 5 units may enable one to add 1, 2 or more grams carbohydrate per unit, but when one is taking 30 units, an added 5 units would have much less effect.

Repeatedly one sees patients who waste insulin. Case No. 11893, supported by the State of Massachusetts, entered the hospital while regularly taking 80–80–80 units, with 5 per cent sugar in the urine. After eight days her weight rose 5 pounds, the sugar in the urine fell to 0.1 per cent, and the total insulin in twenty-four hours instead of 240 units was 50 units.

Insulin should never be omitted when sugar remains in the urine. If vomiting prevents the taking of food, continue the insulin, testing the urine every four hours and only omit a dose when the urine is sugar-free. I know these two sentences are repetitious, but if they are heeded, there will be fewer deaths from diabetic coma. (See pages 155-161.)

Recently, Dr. M. C. Balodimos working with us studied the histories of one hundred patients coming to the Clinic who were taking 80 or more units daily. Of these there was justification for this dosage in a few because of exceptional conditions, but in forty-five it was raised to offset indiscretions in diet. After a few days the diabetes of these patients was controlled with an average of half the former units.

On October 11, 1952, Dr. Janine Duckers found that 68 of our 69 diabetic patients at the New England Deaconess Hospital were taking insulin. Sixty-two were taking NPH or NPH plus RI mixed together, and of these, 29 NPH alone. Six patients were taking PZI. The total dose on this day varied from 10 to 98 units. There were 36 male and 33 female patients. Ages varied from six to eighty-three years.

In general, with protamine zinc insulin one adjusts the diet to the insulin, instead of the insulin into the diet, shifting it from one meal to another or giving it between meals so as to lessen the load for the protamine zinc insulin to carry. The protamine zinc insulin should be increased to bring about a sugar-free specimen on rising and the regular or crystalline insulin increased to keep the urine sugar-free during the waking hours of the day. Sometimes it is advantageous to use NPH insulin both before breakfast and the evening meal.

Having once learned the proper dosage, as a rule one can continue it for months. One would not change the dosage to offset a single day's irregularity in the urinary tests for sugar. Avoid changing diet and insulin on the same day. A change of 10 grams carbohydrate from one time of the day to another may bring not only safety but comfort and a sugar-free urine. One must enlist the patient's cooperation.

Changing from PZI to NPH Insulin

When planning for any change of insulins one should do tests for glycosuria 4 times a day (before meals and at bedtime) for a few days before changing over to the new insulin. The data thus acquired are valuable for comparison when NPH is begun.

With many patients the action of NPH insulin during the forenoon is not rapid and strong enough to prevent blood sugar values at two hours after breakfast from rising to quite high levels. Consequently, with most patients a *forenoon lunch* is unnecessary. Contrariwise, since the peak of NPH action begins in the afternoon, a *mid-afternoon lunch* should be *given uniformly* and, as with all insulins, a bedtime lunch to prevent reactions during the night.

Rule for Giving Insulin When Food is not Retained

Insulin lowers the sugar in the blood and theoretically should always be followed soon by food in order to prevent the sugar in the blood from dropping too low and so producing an insulin reaction. However, if the individual cannot take food and the urine contains sugar, insulin is also indicated because it is proof that sugar is being formed at the expense of the body itself. Under such circumstances insulin should be given every four, six or eight hours, testing the urine before each dose to be sure it is needed. *Never omit insulin unless the urine is sugar-free and the blood sugar normal.* When in doubt consult a physician. Adjust the dose according to the condition of the urine. At the hospital at such times we sometimes write orders

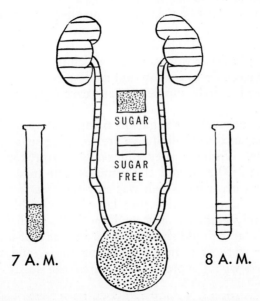

SUGAR

SUGAR FREE

7 A. M.   8 A. M.

Fig. 15.—Sugar may be present in the first specimen voided on rising, but another specimen voided thirty minutes later may be sugar-free. This is because the first specimen represents a mixture of all the urine formed by the kidneys and then passed into the bladder during the night. Although the urine during the first of this period may have contained sugar, it may have been sugar-free in the later period, but the two portions mixing in the bladder conceal what has happened. A second specimen, 30 minutes after the bladder has been emptied, is essential if one wishes to compare urine sugar and blood sugar. Drawn by Sister M. F. T.

as follows: Test urine with Benedict's solution every four hours. If test is red, give 16 units; if orange, give 12 units; if yellow, give 8 units; if green, give 4 units; if no sugar, omit insulin, but repeat the Benedict test every four hours until the patient is able to resume his usual diet and insulin. (See pages 55, 56.) The insulin used in such a condition would be the quick-acting regular or crystalline insulin. Should the patient be under the influence of protamine zinc insulin or the intermediate insulins, smaller doses of crystalline insulin could be prescribed. Always remember that a diabetic patient not eating food is living on his own body—a very, very low carbohydrate, moderate protein but high fat diet; in other words, a diet which does not respond advantageously to insulin and so despite glycosuria, he may need a little supplementary carbohydrate to balance it.

If the urine shows sugar on rising, it does not necessarily mean that the kidneys are secreting sugar at that moment. Perhaps they did secrete urine containing sugar at 2:00 A.M. and the urine became mixed in the bladder with urine which was secreted free from sugar by the kidneys some hours later. If the bladder is completely emptied, a second specimen voided thirty minutes later would show whether in that half-hour the kidneys were or were not secreting sugar, and such a specimen would more nearly match the sugar in the blood.

If a needle breaks and is left under the skin while injecting insulin, do not be alarmed. The needle will not wander. Mark the site by drawing a circle about the point of injection. Draw an arrow in the direction the needle was inserted. Then when a convenient time arrives ask a surgeon and not a doctor like myself to take it out. He will probably desire x-ray pictures to locate it. The removal is not painful, but it is not so easy to find a needle as one might think, indeed, almost as troublesome as to find a gold watch I once lost in my haymow, which Mr. Kay and Jimmie discovered after hours of hard, hot work.

A few patients are allergic to insulin. This is of little importance if of slight degree, because it lasts only temporarily and after a few weeks any local irritation disappears. Rarely benadryl is needed to allay discomfort. If the sensitivity persists, then one must desensitize the patient. This can be done quickly by giving repeated, small doses every half hour or by the use of 1/1000 or 1/10,000 of a unit and doubling the dose at each of four or more injections daily under a doctor's close supervision. No one needs to go without insulin because he is allergic to it.

A patient who has omitted insulin may be allergic to it, if it is resumed after a considerable interval. Consquently, if the doctor allows the omission of insulin, it is desirable to take a token dose of 4 units once a week.

Insulin and an Infection

An infection makes the diabetes more severe. An infection according to Dr. Lukens is Nature's glucose tolerance test and, I would add, pregnancy is too. At such times the insulin must be increased and, as meals are irregular when one is ill, it is often best to increase the number of times insulin has previously been given, so as to take care of all the meals and lunches. If protamine zinc insulin has been employed, continue the regular dose of it and depend upon quick insulin to get control of the diabetes.

During an infection the effect of insulin wears off more quickly. If a patient has been taking 10 units of insulin twice a day (10–0–10), he might need to change to 5 units four times a day (5–5–5–5), or he might increase the dose and alternate between 10 and 5 units every six hours (10–5–10–5). Most likely he would be given a moderate holding dose of PZI, NPH, Globin or Lente insulin before breakfast supplemented by CI, as described on page 55. In pneumonia I have given as much as 100 units a day to a patient with subsequent recovery. Such was Case No. 6762, a street cleaner with chronic asthma. Usually (this was before the discovery of PZI) he injected 20–0–18–2 units of regular insulin, but when he developed pneumonia it rose to 30–30–30–10 units. Three months after discharge from the hospital it fell to 24–0–16 units. A patient during the course of a carbuncle years ago required 100 units in 24 hours, but later none. However, 13 years later she returned with much sugar in her urine!

With another patient, Mrs. G. H. D., aged seventy-one years, the insulin rose from 10 units before the pneumonia to 84 units during it and then fell to 10 units upon recovery. After two trips to Europe she changed to protamine zinc insulin, 12 units once a day. Later she flew to New York and sailed to England for the Coronation in 1937. She was then seventy-four years old, looked the picture of health, took 52 units PZI, could eat about as freely as she liked, but was not quite reconciled to restriction of exercise. Her behavior seemed remarkable in 1937, but now twenty-two years later we see such cases more frequently, so rapidly has progress in treatment advanced.

At present we use NPH insulin for most patients requiring insulin, supplementing it if necessary with crystalline insulin in the morning in the same syringe and more rarely with CI, or exceptionally NPH, again before the evening meal. Crystalline insulin is a purer substance than regular insulin and lasts perhaps an hour longer. Although regular insulin and NPH insulin are the insulins now used by us, if a patient comes to the Clinic doing well with any kind of insulin we are loath to change it. We recognize that occasionally protamine zinc insulin acts more efficiently than NPH.

Protamine zinc insulin, NPH insulin, Lente and Globin insulin to a slightly lesser extent, act during every hour of the day, *"act while you sleep,"* and therefore the body should have in store carbohydrate-forming material to offset their action and prevent hypoglycemia. The long-acting insulins are particularly useful in controlling the diabetes during the sleeping part of the day when the body is without food; the quick-acting insulins supplement control during the eating part of the twenty-four hours. When patients take RI or CI they should eat within thirty minutes.

All insulins are good. By appropriate adjustments of the carbohydrate in the diet, diabetes can be successfully treated by any one variety. When Lente insulin and NPH insulin were used with children at Diabetic Camps, Dr. Marble found actions were practically identical.

Frequent feedings are always useful for the patient taking any insulin and particularly a long-duration insulin, and for several reasons. First, as already said, the lowering of the total carbohydrate at a meal, by the taking away of a small quantity for lunches brings the carbohydrate at that meal to a level which a slow-acting insulin can control. Second, these feedings also protect against the danger of reactions between meals when the blood sugar might be low. Third, it is always advantageous in the administration of carbohydrate to a diabetic to get the benefit which results from the falling tide of a blood-sugar curve, because that decidedly favors the utilization of carbohydrate in contrast to a rising blood-sugar curve which hinders it. Fourth, by promotion of utilization of carbohydrate between meals the development of acidosis is averted. Fifth, frequent feedings of carbohydrate favor its utilization.

INSTRUCTIONS FOR GIVING INSULIN SUBCUTANEOUSLY

1. Sterilizing

Wash the hands thoroughly with soap and water.

Wrap the cylinder and the piston of the syringe separately in a piece of cloth and cover them and the needle with cold water in a dish, heat to boiling, and let boil for five minutes. Pour off the water, being careful not to touch anything in the dish, and allow to cool. One can place syringe and needle in a wire strainer and this in turn in the dish filled with water and thus they can be removed conveniently for cooling at the end of sterilization.

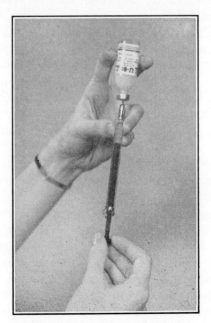

Fig. 16.—Filling a syringe.

Clean the top of the insulin bottle with 70 per cent isopropyl alcohol.

Certain patients, it is true, do not sterilize their syringes and needles by boiling, but by alcohol. I still hesitate to advocate indiscriminately such a method. The hands of the patients who adopt this plan should be exceptionally clean and deft in the handling of syringe and needle.

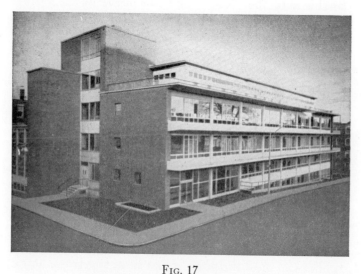

FIG. 17

HOSPITAL TEACHING CLINIC
Operated By
THE NEW ENGLAND DEACONESS HOSPITAL
For
THE DIABETES FOUNDATION, INC.
Boston

To sterilize with alcohol pour the alcohol into a tea-spoon in which the needle has been placed. Wait three minutes. Without inserting fingers into the teaspoon work the syringe into the butt of the needle so that it

10

can be raised from the spoon, and then it can be made fast. Expel the alcohol. Dip the cap of the insulin bottle for sterilization into the spoon containing the alcohol and proceed as usual. After injecting the insulin, draw water through the needle into the syringe and expel it and then draw up alcohol from the teaspoon into the syringe and expel it back and forth into the spoon through the needle and draw air in and out. In this way the plunger and the inside of the syringe are sterilized and ready for the next injection. One can purchase outfits in which syringe and needle can be kept in a tube filled with isopropyl alcohol between injections. There is no objection to keeping syringe and needle in alcohol all the time, but always be careful to avoid any injection of alcohol.

2. Loading

Take barrel and insert the piston into it being careful not to touch the surface of the piston which enters the barrel, and thus contaminate it. Fasten the needle onto the barrel. Draw out the piston so far that the syringe contains a little more air than the amount of insulin needed.

Push the needle cautiously but firmly through the rubber cap until the point is just seen, invert the bottle; force the air from the syringe into the bottle and then withdraw as much insulin as is desired. By holding the syringe and needle point upward, air is easily expelled from the syringe before withdrawing it from the bottle. If cloudy insulin is used, tip the insulin bottle over gently without causing any foam so that when insulin is withdrawn the precipitate will be uniformly distributed.

3. Injecting

The desirable site for injecting insulin is one where the skin is loose. It is imperative to change the place with every dose. Thus the doses can be given in four longitudinal and parallel lines down the extremities and abdomen. The Sunday dose begins at the upper end of each line and the Saturday dose is at the lower end.

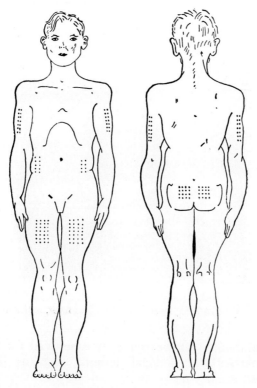

Fig. 18.—Insulin maps.

Never give insulin in two sites within an inch of each other in one month. Necrosis of tissue occurs, an abscess may form, failure of absorption is bound to ensue, the dosage in consequence must be increased, and if by chance this increased quantity is given in another part of the body where absorption is prompt, a reaction follows.

Furthermore, atrophies of the subcutaneous fat may develop and these are quite disfiguring, but never dangerous. In the course of years they may disappear. For such patients, the abdomen and the areas just above the buttocks can be utilized. In our experience it has never been necessary for a patient to give up insulin on account of atrophies. Insulin atrophies are common to both sexes in childhood, but in adults they occur almost exclusively in females.

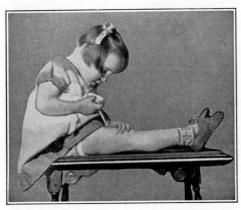

Fig. 19.—Case 9443, aged two years and eleven months, injecting her insulin. Alive in 1959, twenty-seven-years later, and doing well.

The abdomen can be routinely employed for injections, particularly if local lesions, such as insulin atrophies, occur.

Having decided on the site for injection, rub gently an area an inch in diameter with alcohol. Pick up a fold of the skin between the thumb and forefinger of the left hand, and with the syringe held parallel to the skin (not as the little girl in Figure 19) push the needle quickly and firmly into the fold nearly up to the butt. The tip of the needle should then feel loose in the soft tissue between the skin and the muscle.

Force the insulin gradually out of the syringe, while withdrawing the needle slowly, so that all of the insulin may not be left in one spot.

Touch the spot lightly with clean cotton until the insulin has been absorbed.

If the insulin has been given too close to the upper layers of the skin a white blister-like elevation will appear.

Protamine zinc insulin and NPH insulin in their present form are solids. All of their virtue is in the precipitate. Therefore, be sure this is uniformly distributed by gently revolving the bottle.

4. Cleaning Up

Rinse the syringe and needle with cold water immediately. Dry the syringe and needle with a cloth and blow air with the syringe repeatedly through the needle. Rub off any irregularities on the point on a finestone such as a razor hone.

ORAL BLOOD-SUGAR-LOWERING DRUGS

The Sulfonylureas

At the University of Montpellier in Southern France, in 1942, experiments were conducted by Jabon, Loubatieres and their associates upon the efficacy of certain drugs in the treatment of infections. Incidentally, it was noted that symptoms resembling those of an insulin reaction occurred and in fact the blood sugar was found to be low. Extensive clinical application was not made of this observation until 1954, when Franke and Fuchs in Berlin, during their investigations of antibiotics, observed the same phenomenon with a sulfonylurea compound, BZ55. In addition to their research, clinical investigations were undertaken on a large scale by

Bertram in Hamburg, who found that this substance, also known as "Carbutamide," lowered the blood sugar of certain diabetics provided the diabetes was of a milder nature with a low insulin requirement and thus was not the severe, unstable or juvenile type diabetes wholly dependent on insulin.

Although Carbutamide represented a long-wished for drug to replace injections of insulin, it contained no insulin; unlike insulin it was not a constituent of the body; was actually foreign to it and, as yet, no one knows what effect it or other oral blood-sugar-lowering preparations will have if used for years. The sulfonyl-urea drugs do not allow the patient to eat more. Indeed, the diabetes must be controlled even more carefully than with insulin.

Carbutamide had certain undesirable side-effects such as allergic skin rashes and in some instances complications of the liver occurred. However, it was found that by substituting a methyl (CH_3) for an amino (NH_2) group in the para position in the benzene ring, these undesirable effects were eliminated and a second preparation, Tolbutamide, (Orinase) was released in the United States, for general use by physician's prescription, June 10, 1957.

No one claims these oral preparations are the equal of insulin. All agree they should not be used in the presence of complications and should not be given to patients who have controlled their diabetes for 20 or more years with success because, should unusual symptoms arise, one could not tell whether such were caused by the natural course of diabetes or the new drugs. Also, very few patients with long duration diabetes respond satisfactorily to the sulfonylurea drugs.

The technique of treatment with these oral compounds has become simpler and simpler. Gradually, in 2 or 3 days under the close supervision of a physician, insulin is reduced to zero and replaced by 1 to 2 Orinase tablets, one-half gram each, up to a limit of 6 in 24 hours. The dose should be adjusted according to the results of urine and blood sugar tests.

For patients taking a small dose of insulin, 12 units or less, there is another method. Under the direction of a physician omit insulin for 2 days, or change from long-acting to regular or crystalline insulin. The next morning, following a fasting blood sugar test, give 6 Orinase tablets, one-half gram each. From the results of another blood sugar test 4 hours later, if a definite fall in blood sugar level has occurred, one can predict with some certainty whether the drug will be useful to the patient.

Still another drug is Chlorpropamide, (Diabinese.) This also will lower the blood sugar and smaller doses are required. Because it remains longer in the body and excretion in the urine is slower than for Tolbutamide severe insulin-like reactions are possible. Complications such as muscular weakness, skin rashes, digestive disturbances and even jaundice have developed with its use in some patients. This is available by physician's prescription but its use is generally for the same type of patient who responds to Tolbutamide. Its long duration also requires careful watching.

I am more than glad to take advantage of Orinase but as for the other drugs, I depend upon my colleagues now conducting careful studies on their action. This applies also to a fourth drug of this group, Metahexamide, which is at this time on a clinical trial basis only.

The Biguanides

Quite apart from the sulfonylureas is a series of drugs known as Biguanides. Although they do have blood-sugar-lowering qualities they are chiefly of importance in stabilizing the blood sugar in those individuals who have rapid changes from high to low blood sugar values and so are susceptible to reactions. In these patients they are often given with insulin. Some physicians have reported their use in milder diabetics as well. In large doses they sometimes cause digestive upsets. There have been no toxic effects reported in 3000 cases. How important a place the Biguanides which include Phenethylbiguanide (DBI, Phenformin) will fill in the treatment of diabetes is still a question, but at present they should be employed only under the close supervision of a doctor.

They are now available by prescription, but I believe many physicians will not yet desire to use these until more data are available, unless they are in a position to conduct research.

The above statements are made as of May 1, 1959. Progress is so rapid that in the course of 6 months many new facts will appear. Any reader is at liberty to write the author for a revision of the opinions here expressed and gladly a reply will be sent.

Treatment with Exercise (See Chapter 7.)

Exercise is the third horse hitched to the diabetic's chariot and is a great aid to Diet and Insulin. When Exercise works, Diet and Insulin have less to do; the Exercise horse is helping to pull. Exercise will lower the blood sugar and so permits more food and lessens the demand for insulin. A diabetic requires exercise to do well. A patient confined to bed is given bed gymnastics. But one must watch Exercise, because unless one allows for what it does, the blood sugar falls so much below normal that symptoms appear akin to those from an overdose of insulin. The boy who plays hockey, basketball or indulges in any strenuous sport always allows for this and lowers his insulin or raises his carbohydrate, preferably the latter—in other words, adjusts the load for Diet and Insulin. (See pages

77–84.) In a tennis match a diabetic contestant may take a lump of sugar every twenty minutes.

Exercise lessens the requirement for insulin because it lowers the blood sugar. We know this is so because all athletes are so much better off if they take a little carbohydrate during prolonged exercise to prevent their blood sugar becoming too low. The same holds true of a mild diabetic; exercise lowers his blood sugar. *But it is entirely different with a severe diabetic.* He is made worse with exercise unless he makes himself like a normal individual by taking enough insulin to compensate for what his pancreas fails to produce and thus be able to utilize carbohydrate calories and not live entirely on fat calories. If he does this, exercise helps him, too.

Anyone using insulin of any type should have an extra 5 to 20 grams of carbohydrate handy if he undertakes unusual exercise. Of course if he knows about this in advance, he might lessen his insulin, but I think it safer for him to take the additional food; particularly true is this for those using protamine zinc insulin or the intermediate insulins. With protamine zinc insulin he may need a second supply of food, because protamine zinc insulin acts longer. In fact, the diabetic, when taking an adequate dosage of insulin, almost resembles a normal individual and yet may be lacking in carbohydrate (glycogen) in his body and therefore, just like the healthy athlete, requires extra food.

Naunyn's Principles of Treatment[1]

"Although the course of the disease is by no means exclusively dependent upon glycosuria, yet it is the important symptom, because in general its severity gives the single reliable measure by which the severity of the disease can be measured, and because in and of itself it carries many dangers. This surely holds true for the higher grades of glycosuria. These always bring

[1] Naunyn: Der Diabetes Melitus, Wien, Holder, pp. 256–258, 1898.

to the patient, earlier or later, serious danger through exhaustion and dangerous complications.

"The glycosuria shows in many cases of diabetes an outspoken tendency to progression; in the majority of cases this tendency to progression is only an expression of the bad influence which it, the glycosuria itself, exerts on the tolerance.

"Each severe glycosuria in a diabetic ought permanently to be prevented since it will sooner or later become threatening; indeed the glycosuria ought to be banished on account of the favorable influence which the aglycosuric condition exerts on the tolerance. Unconditionally, this must be attempted at the beginning of treatment.

"Above all it is important for the first traces of the diabetes to be energetically treated at their first appearance in order that, if possible, the conquest of the glycosuria may be obtained. I consider it in my experience very probable that among the early strenuously treated cases, which in the beginning imposed themselves as being very severe but later on ran a favorable course there is many a one for which this very early, strict treatment is responsible, and on the other hand there can be no doubt that the end result of the milder cases, which late if ever were energetically treated, was in the majority of instances that they became severe.

"I consider it a pessimistic curtailment of the task resting on the doctor in the treatment of diabetes if it is said 'the essential task of the doctor is and remains to maintain the patient for a long time in a bearable condition of life.' According to my view the treatment has a broader and more definite purpose, namely this: to better the disturbed function or at least to prevent its further deterioration, the progressive development of the disease. It is understood on the other hand that it is allowed transitorily to undernourish the patient provided thereby it is only in this way possible to obtain control of the disease."

11

DIABETIC COMA

DIABETIC coma (acid intoxication, acidosis, ketosis) used to be the nightmare of doctor and patient. Before 1914, two-thirds of our diabetic patients and nearly all diabetic children succumbed to it. Treatment by undernutrition lowered the coma deaths to about forty-two per cent. Since the introduction of insulin in 1922, deaths from diabetic coma have continued to decrease until now they approach one per cent. Among carefully treated diabetics it can be completely avoided. Statistics on the reduction in mortality from diabetic coma in my own practice were compiled for me by the Metropolitan Life Insurance Company. The percentage of coma deaths compared to all deaths of diabetics is shown in Figure 20.

This fall in mortality is due first to the prevention of the causes which lead to coma and second to insulin. Above all else remember that diabetic coma comes on like a thief in the night. Whenever a diabetic feels sick, he should call it coma and follow the rules given on page 157. Coma is most frequent in childhood, because in childhood diabetes is usually more severe and more dependent upon insulin, but it is most fatal in adults who cannot withstand its catastrophic onslaught. Prompt treatment is nearly always successful.

The acid intoxication which develops in a diabetic resembles that which develops in a normal individual when he stops eating carbohydrate. Under such circumstances when there is no carbohydrate to burn in the body or what amounts to the same thing in diabetes when the body cannot burn it, because of lack of in-

(155)

sulin, the body must draw on fat for nourishment and if that is eaten in excess, fat ceases to be burned completely and fatty acids multiply. These fatty acids are poisonous, cause acid poisoning (ketosis) and, unless removed from the body or completely burned up in it may lead to diabetic coma and death.

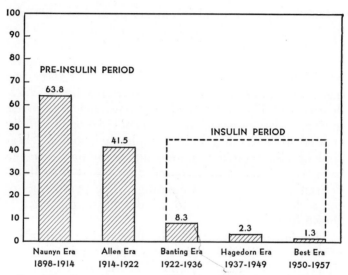

Fig. 20.—Coma as a cause of death. Percentage of all deaths due to diabetic coma. Percentages Prepared by the Statistical Department of the Metropolitan Life Insurance Company.

The invariable cause of acid poisoning is well understood. It is due to lack of insulin and when this occurs then carbohydrate ceases to be burned and the body is forced to live on so much fat that it cannot assimilate it and acid poisoning (ketosis) results. Overeating brings it on because it makes the diabetes more severe. Overeating can lead to death by coma. It makes no difference whether the overeating comes from food (breaking the diet) or whether it comes from an infection which also makes the diabetes more severe and at the same time, because of the accompanying fever, burns up the tissues more rapidly. Indeed the latter condition is the more serious. Overeating of food is easily corrected, but overeating of one's own body as in pneumonia and similar infections is controlled with difficulty, and for most diabetics only with insulin. Inflammatory conditions and certain types of goiter likewise lead to an increased metabolism, *i.e.*, overeating of the body, but most of these states may be relieved by surgery, or medication.

TREATMENT OF ACID INTOXICATION

Rules for the Patient

1. Send for the doctor, at the same time reporting the condition of the urine.

2. Go to bed.

3. Liquids. A cupful an hour. Hot water, tea, coffee, broths, beef tea, clear soups and water oatmeal gruel.

4. Take an enema. The enema clears the lower intestine so that salt solution, a teaspoonful of salt to each pint of water, can be given later by the rectum in case liquids are not retained by mouth and opportunity is not available to take them subcutaneously or by vein, which latter method is by far the more preferable and usual.

5 Keep warm: woolen blankets, flannel night-clothes, heaters, but put a blanket about the heater to avoid burns.

6. Secure a nurse or someone in the family who will spend the entire time caring for you until the doctor arrives, or says you are out of danger. Recovery (partial or complete) or death usually occurs within the first forty-eight hours.

7. Do not omit insulin if urine shows sugar.

Questions for the Doctor

1. Has this patient acidosis and is it severe enough to

account for the present symptoms? Is an insulin reaction excluded?

2. If so, how much and how frequently is clear (regular or crystalline) insulin to be given? Twenty, 30, 40,
50, 100 or more units? Every half hour or every hour?
What does the urine or blood indicate?

3. Is the patient dry? Does he not need immediately
1, 2 or more quarts of salt solution injected intravenously or perhaps subcutaneously?

4. Is the stomach dilated? Does it demand lavage to
hasten the time when the patient can take and retain
nourishment? In nine cases out of ten, we wash out the
stomach to prevent the patient later regurgitating food
into the lungs.

5. Is there a lack of potassium? This may occur in
prolonged coma or when the patient has been given
carbohydrate, which carries it with potassium into the
cells. An analysis of the blood or electrocardiogram
may disclose it.

6. Does the heart need caffeine sodium benzoate, $7\frac{1}{2}$
grains in repeated doses, or other stimulation? We
think the best stimulant for the heart is the replacement
of loss of liquid by intravenous salt solution given slowly.

In the convalescence, patient and physician, too, will
do well to make haste slowly. Carbohydrate up to 50
grams, however, should be given and retained and absorbed by the patient during the first twelve hours of
active treatment if the blood sugar is falling, and during
the next twelve hours at least as much more. This will
suffice for temporary nutrition with the gradual addition of protein and fat as rapidly as the stomach will
bear food. If carbohydrate is not retained, when given
by mouth, 25, 50 or even 100 grams of glucose must be
given intravenously or subcutaneously during the first
24 hours of treatment, but we never give glucose until
the blood sugar is approaching a normal value.

It is a shame for a diabetic patient to die of diabetic

coma, because coma is practically always preventable. Patients must keep their diabetes under control to avoid coma and this means that no days should go by without at least one or more of the specimens voided being sugar-free. I will admit that with the diets higher in carbohydrate than formerly and with greater activity upon the part of the patients this is more difficult, but it can be done and should be done, if one wishes to be free from serious degenerative disease after twenty-five years of diabetes.

There are simple tests for disclosing the presence of acid poisoning in the urine. Such are Acetest but I prefer a sugar-free urine.

Recovery from coma should be sure, provided a good laboratory is available from start to finish. We thought our results good when our hospital mortality for actual coma dropped to 14 per cent, but it fell to 1.2 per cent when the same amount of insulin, about 250 units, was given earlier in the first three hours of treatment instead of in the first twelve hours. For such rapid administration, blood sugar determinations in a laboratory are invaluable, because they are the guide to dosage of insulin. Recently in two large hospitals 133 cases were treated in succession without a death.

There is always a reason for diabetic coma and the reason is overeating of food or overeating of the body and diabetics should never forget this fact. For the overeating of fat of the body, which accompanies an infection or an overactive thyroid, (hyperthyroidism) the patient is blameless, but for the overeating of food he is responsible. Since an infection always makes the diabetes more severe, the patient should be prepared to meet it by increasing insulin, or, if not taking it regularly, being ready to employ it. Never omit insulin so long as the urine contains sugar.

A sugar-free urine spells safety for a diabetic. A sugar-free urine implies that he is not overeating, and it is from overeating, from taking more fat than can be burned that acid intoxication results. Danger from acid poisoning vanishes in 999 cases out of 1000 if a diabetic is sugar-free. A given amount of fat may be utilized or burned up, but if too much is given either from the food or from the body it cannot be used up and consequently appears in the urine as acid bodies—the acetone (ketone) bodies.

Before the discovery of insulin, deaths from acid poisoning decreased with the advent of undernutrition, the reverse of overeating. In my practice this was accomplished by the restriction of fat, which is so rich in calories. However, although cases ceased to originate in hospitals while under a doctor's eye, that did not protect all diabetics.

Insulin and undernutrition both help carbohydrate to burn, and with the burning of carbohydrate in the body, there is less necessity to draw on an excess of fat for maintenance and then acidosis vanishes like dew before the sun. Therefore, no wonder there are fewer cases of diabetic coma today. There need be none if care is taken in the diet and insulin is used in season. On the other hand, if the patient has been taking a diet more than would be possible for him to take and keep sugar-free without the use of insulin and then suddenly omits his insulin and continues to eat the same amount of food, diabetic coma can occur with surprising swiftness. A diabetic taking insulin is walking on insulin stilts. Take away the stilts and he falls. Never omit insulin when sugar is present in the urine even if you are not eating or retaining food. Under such circumstances even sugar formed by the breakdown of protein in the body is lost because a severe diabetic, unlike a normal individual, cannot sufficiently utilize it and he is compelled to live on fat.

A diabetic boy overeats at Thanksgiving on Thursday. If he breaks his diet that day it is fairly good evidence he has broken it before. Upon Friday and Saturday he may have indigestion and vomiting. Not caring for food perhaps he neglects insulin and feels "sick." He is irritable, thirsty, but does not keep down the food he takes; his bowels are neglected. He feels weak and loses interest, becomes sleepy and stuporous and breathes heavily with air hunger. Before anyone realizes the fact unconsciousness develops and only the miracle working action of insulin will save him.

Signs of the Onset of Acid Poisoning; Its Prevention and Early Treatment.

The symptoms and signs of diabetic coma are most indefinite. Consequently, it is a good rule for any diabetic patient if he feels "sick," and has nausea, vomiting or pain in the abdomen, and always if he has fever, to take for granted that he may have acid posioning and adopt those measures which will prevent its becoming serious. These are very simple, and are as follows:

When approaching or in diabetic coma the safest place for the patient is in a hospital. Diabetics should think in advance to which hospital they wish to go in case of an accident, diabetic coma or an insulin reaction.

There is another angle to the diabetic coma situation which Dr. Priscilla White found when she analyzed its incidence in our diabetic children. Diabetic coma is an index of adherence to good treatment or to its neglect. Thus, of 220 children and young adults who had had coma repeatedly, the prevalence of an incapacitating arteriosclerosis in the eyes, heart, kidneys, brain or blood vessels generally was 58 per cent; but in those who were free from vascular disease only 10 per cent had ever had coma.

12

THE DIFFERENCES BETWEEN DIABETIC COMA AND INSULIN REACTIONS

DIABETIC coma is due to acid poisoning, is serious, and if untreated leads to death. It is caused by lack of insulin, due to overeating, often by breaking the diet, especially by omitting the insulin which has made eating the regular meals safe, or it may occur when the patient overeats of himself as in the course of fever and infections or in some kinds of goiter. Coma is preventable and curable. (See page 155).

Coma implies too little insulin or uncontrolled diabetes. An insulin reaction is the opposite. Often it is caused by injecting too much insulin, unusual exercise, insufficient food or lessening of the severity of the diabetes.

An insulin reaction is explained by the blood sugar falling too low. This may be due to too much insulin, to the taking of too little food after the injection of insulin or its poor absorption due to vomiting and diarrhea, or to so much exercise that the food eaten has been used up, and the sugar in the blood has dropped too low. Although insulin reactions almost never cause death, they can do so if not recognized and can be serious, because they may occur in places where they are embarrassing or dangerous to the patient. They can be prevented by taking a little carbohydrate to raise the sugar in the blood to normal when the first warning signal appears or, better still, by a little food between meals and upon retiring, and in this way avoiding a low blood sugar.

For several years one patient had had no reactions, but when diarrhea lasted four days during a summer vacation a reaction came while he was repairing his canoe.

Another patient worked in a ship-building plant. Of a Saturday morning his wife asked him to polish the kitchen floor. This he started to do, but the woman's customary work was so much more strenuous than the man's daily work that he developed a reaction. The following week the problem was solved by his wife adding a small doughnut to his breakfast.

TABLE 10.—DIABETIC COMA AND INSULIN SHOCK—
DIFFERENTIAL DIAGNOSIS

	Diabetic Coma	Insulin Shock
1. Onset	Slow—days	Sudden—minutes
2. Food	Too much	Too little
3. Insulin	Too little	Too much
4. Presence of infection	Frequent	None
5. Thirst	Extreme	Absent
6. Hunger	Absent	Frequent
7. Nausea and vomiting	Common	Seldom, except with protamine zinc insulin
8. Pain in abdomen	Frequent	Absent
9. Fever	Absent except with infection	Absent
10. Skin	Dry	Moist
11. Tremor	Absent	Frequent
12. Vision	Dim	Double
13. Eyeballs	Soft	Normal
14. Appearance	Florid—extremely ill	Pale—weak—faint
15. Respiration	Air-hunger	Normal
16. Blood-pressure	Tends to fall	Tends to rise
17. Mental state	Restless—distressed	Headache—apathetic—irritable—hysterical
18. Unconsciousness	Gradually approaches	May intervene suddenly
19. Urine: sugar	Present	Absent (always in 2d specimen)
20. Urine: diacetic acid and acetone	Present	Absent
21. Blood: sugar	High	Low
22. Specific treatment	Insulin—fluid—salt	Carbohydrate
23. Response to treatment	Gradual—hours	Quick—minutes

A diabetic should never drive an automobile for more than two hours without taking a little carbohydrate, *e.g.*, an orange or its equivalent, in order to guard against his blood sugar becoming too low. A clergyman forgetting to do this, while candidating for a new parish, landed in the town jail instead of in the town pulpit.

Diabetic coma is always avoidable by following the rules of treatment. An insulin reaction may occur accidentally, but is usually preventable.

One of the reasons I cannot advise the use of alcohol by diabetics is the danger of an insulin reaction being unrecognized if the breath shows a trace of an alcoholic odor. I have a high estimation of policemen; they make reliable patients, but it is unreasonable to expect that there will always be a diabetic sergeant in every station-house ready to detect an insulin reaction or diabetic coma when the individual is arrested and supposed to be drunk.

Protamine zinc insulin and the intermediate insulins cause reactions, but they are usually less severe although more prolonged and, unlike those due to regular or crystalline insulin, are frequently accompanied by nausea, sometimes vomiting, and headache. These symptoms make the differential diagnosis between reactions from the longer-acting insulins and coma more difficult than that between reactions from regular or crystalline insulin and coma. Reactions from regular insulin most commonly occur in the late morning or early afternoon, but from protamine zinc insulin they appear in the late afternoon, evening or night, and from NPH, Lente and Globin insulin in the late afternoon. A reaction due to regular insulin is usually relieved by taking a little carbohydrate once, but when due to protamine zinc insulin, it may be necessary to repeat it in an hour. If a patient does not show definite signs of recovery from a supposed insulin reaction, and this applies to diabetic coma as well, in fifteen minutes, he should be transferred to a hospital where a laboratory is available.

Treatment of an Insulin Reaction

The quickest treatment is the injection of 10 or more grams carbohydrate (glucose) intravenously. It is worth while today for a doctor to carry a 20 cc. ampoule of 50 per cent glucose in his bag, because there are now so many diabetics employed in active occupations. If glucose is not available, a carbohydrate drink—Coca Cola—or any liquid containing two teaspoonfuls of sugar should be given. A lump of sugar or a teaspoonful of Karo syrup may be inserted inside the cheek. Don't pour liquid into the mouth of an unconscious patient. Unless recovery occurs promptly and always within half and hour, the patient should be hospitalized, because further treatment requires all the resources of a chemical laboratory.

Relief from an insulin reaction is usually obtained promptly, provided treatment is not delayed. If the reaction is severe, doctors occasionally train the relatives of their patients to give 0.3 to 0.5 of 1 cc. of 1 to 1000 solution adrenalin subcutaneously. Occasionally an injection of diluted glucose into the vein by the doctor is required. For emergencies when out of reach of a physician, as upon a camping trip, especially prepared 10 per cent glucose in 20 cc. ampoules can be injected under the skin by a relative or nurse, but recourse to such a procedure has been needed with only one of our patients. It has been a real comfort to many patients, however, to know that they had with them outfits for the subcutaneous injection of glucose. Each hour the insulin reaction lasts after its onset, the more difficult is recovery.

When insulin has been injected many times into the same area and a lump has formed then absorption is delayed. If the same dose is injected into a fresh area an insulin reaction may occur.

Identification Card

It is desirable for a diabetic to carry in his pocket an identification card. One of my patients wears a bracelet upon the inside of which is inscribed, in addition to his name and address, the words:

COMA OR INSULIN SHOCK. WHICH?

Another patient in her handbag has a metal sign with the words:

I AM A DIABETIC

One of my patients has a 105 per cent wife, but one January she came in worried and wondered what had happened to her husband. He did not want to get up in the morning, was hard to rouse and cross, and yet she realized his diabetes was getting milder, because he was sugar-free despite the protamine zinc insulin being reduced from 36 to 28 units. Why? She had *overlooked* the fact that he had recently taken up curling on the ice, which involved considerable *exercise*—and exercise lowers the blood sugar.

Mary climbed the White Mountains without harm for three days with her professional father. The next day she returned home, took her insulin as usual and lay down for an afternoon nap but woke up in a hospital. The good effects of her strenuous exercise had persisted and her usually close observation of her condition had been relaxed. Her blood sugar had fallen to a reaction level. After twenty-five years of diabetes she had a healthy baby and here he is in Fig. 21, together with his brother, born two years later, after her twenty-seven years of diabetes and her third child born after thirty-one years of diabetes. Mary is Number 24 Victory Medal Case

The same week a devoted couple arrived and the story was that the fond husband on returning from a business trip was wretched, showed more sugar, but also was so cross that his wife threatened to tell his

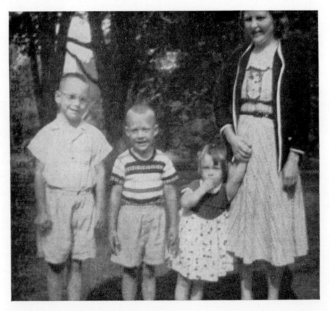

Fig. 21

sister. The wife finally solved the riddle by finding in her husband's bag a new insulin bottle which showed while away he had *bought regular* insulin *instead of his customary protamine zinc* insulin.

A college student ended an important examination with the thought that his mind did not work as well as it should and that he probably would receive a C instead of an A upon the theory that his blood sugar was low.

Perhaps he was correct, but I do know that he should have had 3 lumps of sugar on his desk with his watch and taken one hourly, just as Richardson during a tennis match may take a lump of sugar every twenty minutes. (See Fig. 12, p. 82.) Furthermore, at the end of the examination he could have secured a blood-sugar test which, if it haply proved to be at an insulin reaction level, might have protected his scholarship in the eyes of the authorities.

No college student can afford to go without a careful medical check-up at least once a month. Without it he or she cannot expect us to intervene in his or her behalf if scholastic difficulties arise. And remember for insurance or for employment a letter from a doctor showing a patient is controlling his diabetes is invaluable.

"We are spinning our own fates, good or evil, and never to be undone. Every smallest stroke of virtue or of vice leaves its ever so little scar. The drunken Rip Van Winkle, in Jefferson's play, excuses himself for every fresh dereliction by saying, 'I won't count this time!' Well! he may not count it, and a kind Heaven may not count it; but it is being counted none the less. Down among his nerve cells and fibres the molecules are counting it, registering and storing it up to be used against him when the next temptation comes. Nothing we ever do is, in strict scientific literalness, wiped out."

From *As William James Said:*
*A Treasury of His Work**

*Ed., Elizabeth Perkins Aldrich, The Vanguard Press, New York, 1942.

13

AN INSULIN SYRINGE

It is a good rule, when you visit a doctor, to show him your insulin syringe and insulin bottle.

The American Diabetes Association recommends a syringe graduated in units according to whether the insulin is of U-40 or U-80 strength. Our custom has been to use a one cubic centimeter syringe divided into ten parts and then each part would contain 4 to 8 units, depending upon the strength of the insulin, 40 or 80 units to one cubic centimeter.

Two strengths of insulin are now on the market— U-40 and U-80 insulin. These labels mean that U-40 insulin (red label) has 40 units in one cubic centimeter and U-80 insulin (green label) has 80 units in one cubic centimeter, which is the capactiy of most syringes.

Some syringes contain 1 cubic centimeter, but instead of being subdivided and designated as tenths of a cubic centimeter are marked in units for the convenience of the patient. Upon one side of the scale the units are given for the use of U-40 insulin; upon the other side of the scale for the stronger U-80 insulin. This avoids the necessity of calculations, but the patient must be careful and read the strength of the insulin printed upon the label on his bottle and then use the corresponding scale of the syringe. As a matter of fact the syringes are always divided into 10 parts.

The strength of insulin used does not change the insulin dosage. The prescribed dose in units remains the same, but if one used U-80 insulin, one would inject half the volume which would be necessary to get the same number of units if one employed U-40 insulin.

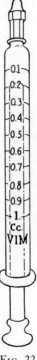

Do not blunder. Be sure you know how much insulin you are taking. The sooner you learn how to give yourself insulin, the better.

This syringe holds 40 units if filled full with U-40 insulin up to the mark 1, and 4 units if filled to the mark 0.1. If it is filled with U-80 insulin it contains 80 units and 8 units at the 0.1 mark.

Fɪɢ. 22.

Be careful! Some syringes hold 2 centimeters instead of one.

14

CARE OF THE TEETH

IT IS regrettable that the teeth of adult diabetic patients are often very poor, but this high incidence is no greater than in non-diabetic patients. It is encouraging that there are so many young diabetics who are comparatively free from dental disease. The period of greatest susceptibility to caries in the teeth is between the ages of seven and twenty. The destruction of teeth and the supporting structures is unusually active just prior to the recognition and treatment of diabetes. If diabetes begins before the age of nine years, there is a good chance that the patients can retain their teeth and have healthy mouths, presumably because treatment is prompt.

In patients with diabetic coma the mucous membranes of the mouth are usually dehydrated and have a dull cherry-red appearance. The teeth may become loose during and immediately following coma, but tighten when the diabetes is brought under control.

It is not difficult to understand why a patient with uncontrolled diabetes of long standing should be susceptible to dental caries and pyorrhea. Added to the influence of acidosis and dehydration there is the factor of lowered resistance to infection which occurs in uncontrolled diabetes. With this and with lowered vitality of tissue, the gums may become unhealthy, pyorrhea and absorption of the alveolar soft tissue may take place and peridental infection develop. However, with proper treatment and control of the diabetic condition the teeth and gums remain in as good condition as those of a non-diabetic person.

Although tartar deposits, gingivitis and pyorrhea may be found in the mouths of adult patients whose diabetes is controlled, these changes are not as progressive as in those patients with poorly controlled diabetes. In the well-controlled group the susceptibility to caries seems low. The teeth can be removed or minor operations performed in the mouth without fear of complications.

At the present time, using insulin if necessary, it is possible to allow adequate diets which are the equal or the superior of average, unselected diets in their completeness. It is possible, and indeed necessary, to include milk and other dairy products in the dietary of every diabetic, young and old. To insure an adequate calcium intake the diet of every adult diabetic should contain at least 0.7 gram of calcium per day and that of every juvenile diabetic 1 gram of calcium a day. See page 118. By this means and by the liberal use of sunlight, cod-liver oil and foods containing vitamin C, one can hope to build and maintain strong teeth and bones.

There is another reason why good treatment of diabetes should automatically include proper care of the teeth. Perhaps more than any other large group of individuals in the country, diabetics visit their doctors often and have frequent physical examinations. If both doctor and patient are alert to their responsibilities, early dental defects are noted and treatment instituted before irreparable damage is done.

Bad teeth are worse than no teeth and are a handicap to a diabetic because the infection which accompanies them makes the diabetes worse. A diabetic cannot afford to tolerate anything which makes his disease more severe. Consequently he should get rid of all the poor teeth which treatment cannot save. So important do we believe this to be that a dental hygienist examines the teeth of all hospital diabetic patients and makes a preliminary report to the dentist who later advises as to treatment or extraction.

Time spent in a hospital by a diabetic to get sugar-free and learn the diet should be utilized to have the teeth put into perfect condition. Such patients receive individual instruction in the method of home care and all our patients may consult the dentist or dental hygienist about his or her dental problems.

CARE OF THE MOUTH AND TEETH

1. Invariably rinse the mouth with water after a meal to remove all food particles.

2. Use a small toothbrush with tufts well separated. Have two brushes and alternate each time you brush your teeth. Replace brush when bristles become soft.

3. A mixture of equal quantities of bicarbonate of soda and table salt is a satisfactory tooth powder.

4. Brush your teeth at least twice daily, morning and night, spending two minutes each time. Be sure that you do this properly. Ask the dental hygienist to show you how if you are not sure.

5. After brushing the teeth, massage the gums with your fingers, working fingers toward the teeth in a rotary motion. This is particularly important for diabetics.

6. Have your teeth cleaned and examined by a dentist or dental hygienist every three months. Keep all cavities filled.

Dr. E. J. Durling has outlined the rules followed at the dental clinic at the New England Deaconess Hospital regarding extractions.

1. The diabetic condition of the patient should be under good control.

2. Local anesthesia, as with novocaine, is preferable since this does not necessitate omission of food prior to its administration or does it interfere with the scheduled

use of insulin. Novocaine, containing the least amount of adrenalin necessary for the operation, is preferable to avoid undesirable blood sugar shifts.

3. The technique used should be as nearly aseptic as possible.

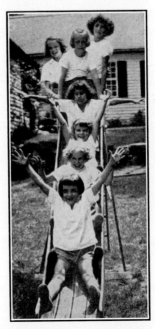

FIG. 23.—Happy diabetic children at play at the Clara Barton Birthplace Camp for diabetic girls.

4. Care should be taken to minimize injury to the gums and with this in mind only a few teeth should be extracted at one time.

5. To avoid postoperative bleeding, all sockets or wounds should be carefully sutured.

6. Consideration should be given to the use of penicillin at a suitable interval prior to the extraction, especially in cases of infection.

One of the advantages to the patient in having a chronic disease like diabetes is the detailed attention the body receives from the physician. The neuritis and pains in various parts of the body which used to be attributed to diabetes were probably often independent of the disease and brought on by other causes, such as the deficient and improperly balanced diets, which were the rule, or smouldering infections. The health examination which a diabetic should receive at each visit should protect him against many ills which non-diabetics thoughtlessly acquire.

We have found that when an adult diabetic has his teeth and gums examined every three months, when he takes the proper home care of the mouth, when his diabetes is under control and is checked by a physician frequently, he has a good chance to retain his teeth as long as a non-diabetic.

15

GANGRENE, INFECTIONS OF THE SKIN

The diabetic should be the cleanest person in the community.

Gangrene

Patients live three times as long with their diabetes and are twenty years older when they die than a generation ago. Gangrene is a disease of older people and is associated with hardening of the arteries. It is most encouraging therefore, that it has decreased from 8 per cent to 2.2 per cent as a cause of death of diabetics. This is due to better care of the feet, better surgery, sulfa drugs and antibiotics and the special attention our patients have received from our friends the chiropodists. Proof of this lies in the fact that fatalities from other sites of hardening of the arteries (arteriosclerosis), which represent the aging process, in the same time advanced. Nevertheless gangrene exacts a dreadful toll from diabetes. In Boston alone, Dr. Root could show diabetic gangrene cost more than one million dollars a year. Patients lost about 4 to 6 weeks between the date of injury and entrance to the hospital; they remain in the hospital another 4 to 6 weeks; on discharge they require a further 4 to 6 weeks to convalesce.

Gangrene is much more common in diabetics than in non-diabetics. No diabetic expects to get gangrene or having gangrene to die of it. The overwhelming majority of all such deaths are needless and could be avoided by cleanliness, proper care of the feet, and early treatment of all wounds, insignificant though they are in the beginning. Exceptionally gangrene will develop because of the closure of a blood vessel and without any previous injury. Cleanliness is here not a factor. Each patient treated at the Deaconess Hospital is told to protect the reputation of the institution and its doctors and his own reputation as well through avoiding death by gangrene.

Gangrene is common in the old, rare in the young. The average age for the development of gangrene in our series is sixty-four years, the youngest thirty-two years and the oldest eighty-nine years. It comes because the circulation in the legs is poor. In only five instances have we noted gangrene in an upper extremity. The legs are far from the heart, and the blood must return uphill; the legs are used much, their blood vessels wear out, especially when they are compelled to carry 200 pounds day after day, and gangrene occurs particularly in those who have been fat. Amputations of an extremity are far less frequent today because of the modern transmetatarsal (partial removal of the toes) operation introduced by Dr. Leland S. McKittrick. Today also, amputations are sometimes avoided by grafting a new blood vessel to replace an occluded one. It is astonishing to see what modern surgery makes possible.

Gangrene and infections of the feet requiring operation are especially common in fat diabetics. Dr. Root reports that of 170 patients undergoing transmetatarsal operations, in 22 cases the average maximum weight was 245 pounds; in 52, 208 pounds; and in 50, 170 pounds. In only 4 cases was the maximum weight under 150 pounds.

Gangrene becomes more frequent the longer the diabetic lives. Each added year of diabetes exposes him more to gangrene. This is easily explained. Gangrene results from poor circulation, and one's circulation is more and more impaired as age advances. This applies to non-diabetics as well as to diabetics and here we are up against a stone wall. The second reason in a measure is being overcome. Hitherto diabetics grew old faster than non-diabetics, but with the introduction of insulin,

12

which has allowed more carbohydrate and less fat in the diet, diabetics age less rapidly and there is no question in my mind but that the carefully treated diabetic is thus helped to retain his youth. Whether the reduction of animal fats in the diet will lessen arteriosclerosis awaits proof.

Unless complicated by a sudden occlusion of a vessel by a blood clot or the results of an infection, gangrene comes on slowly with few symptoms. Increasing inability to walk even for a short distance without pain (intermittent claudication) may go on for weeks or years. Pain at night in the leg, while at rest in bed even without any ulceration, and cramps in the leg are not infrequent, and may be avoided by walking about the room before retiring and lying down for several short periods during the evening. Numbness, tingling and prickling of the toes, coldness of the feet, and sensitiveness to cold weather are premonitory symptoms that the circulation in an extremity is deficient. Sleeping with the legs extended straight and with bed socks may give relief. Control of the diabetes is important.

Physical examination may show a change in temperature by passing the hand downwards from the thighs. Pulsations in the blood vessels of the feet may be absent. If raised, the foot becomes markedly pale but when dependent for a minute becomes red and congested. Atrophy of the muscles and skin may be present and pigmented areas and scars remaining from old yet minor injuries. Calcification of the blood vessels disclosed by *x*-ray is not necessarily a sign of poor circulation.

A Beauty Parlor for Diabetic Feet

The prevalence of complications in the feet of diabetics with the prolonged hospital stay which it involved led to the establishment of what we called first the Beauty Parlor for Diabetic Feet at the New England Deaconess Hospital, but now is an office for the chiropodist and the two "special" foot nurses. Here our diabetic patients are taught the care of the feet so as to avoid gangrene. Dr. John Kelly, an officer in the American Chiropody Association, joined us in 1928, and has spread the knowledge of the vulnerability of the feet of diabetics among chiropodists and their diabetic clients throughout the United States. The chiropodists are our greatest allies in the prevention of gangrene. Many hospitals today have a chiropodist attached to their staffs. To them I gladly accord credit in the campaign for the reduction of mortality due to gangrene.

TREATMENT OF THE FEET

Hygiene of the Feet

1. Wash feet daily with soap and tepid water. Dry thoroughly and gently, especially between toes.

2. When thoroughly dry, rub with lanolin if necessary to keep the skin soft, free from scales and dryness, but never render the feet tender.

3. If nails are brittle and dry, soften by soaking in warm water one-quarter hour each night for a few nights and apply lanolin generously under and about nails and bandage loosely. Clean nails with orangewood sticks. Cut the nails only in a good light and after a bath, when the feet are clean. Cut nails straight across. If you go to a chiropodist, tell him you have diabetes.

4. All patients with overlapping toes or toes that are close together should separate them by lamb's wool. Patients with large joints or cramped-up toes should wear shoes without box toes and only vici kid leather.

5. All patients over sixty should have daily rest periods and remove their shoes. Every Sunday morning ask someone to examine your feet.

6. Do not wear bedroom slippers when you ought to wear shoes. Slippers do not give proper support. Do not step on floor with bare feet, a common source of injury and infection.

7. Wear shoes of soft leather which fit and are not tight (neither narrow nor short). Wear new shoes one-half hour only on the first few nights after purchase.

8 Use bed socks for warmth but *no hot-water bottles, bags or electric heaters and don't put the feet in the oven! Don't burn the feet!* Electric blankets are harmless.

9. After fifty years of age one hears less well, sees less well, and the sense of feeling is diminished. Remember this and be cautious about the feet. A diabetic may walk all day with a nail penetrating his foot and not feel any pain. Indeed this sign of lack of sensation (neuritis) is a most important factor in gangrene.

Treatment of Corns and Callosities

Corns and calluses are dangerous because the skin over them may be broken and infection result. The circulation is so poor in them that healing occurs with difficulty. Hard corns occur chiefly on the external surface of the fifth toes. Soft corns occur between the toes and are a result of ringworm, athlete's foot—epidermophytosis. Plantar warts are of a different nature and should be treated only by those with wide experience.

1. Wear shoes which fit and cause no pressure.

2. For cleanliness soak foot in warm, not hot, soapy water. Rub off dead skin on or about callus or corn with gauze, emery board, fine pumice stone or file. Do not tear it off. Do not cut corns or callosities. Do not try to remove corns or calluses with patent or other medicines.

I have only once heard a surgeon at the New England Deaconess Hospital tell a patient to soak *sore* feet in water or in water to which Epsom salts or any kind of antiseptic had been added. (Temporarily this might be done in the hospital under supervision of a nurse.) Bed rest and dry dressings are the essentials.

3. Prevent calluses under ball of foot. (*a*) by exercise, such as curling and stretching toes twenty times a day, (*b*) by finishing each step on the toes and not on the ball of the foot.

Aids in Treatment of Imperfect Circulation—Cold Feet

1. Exercises. Bend the foot down and up as far as it will go six times. Describe a circle to the left with the foot six times and then to the right. Repeat morning, noon and night.

Buerger's Passive Exercises.[1]—"The affected limb is elevated with the patient lying in bed, to from 60 to 90 degrees above the horizontal, being allowed to rest upon a support for thirty seconds to three minutes. the period of time being the minimum amount necessary to produce blanching or ischemia. As soon as blanching is established, the patient allows the foot to hang down over the edge of the bed for from two to five minutes, until reactionary hyperemia or rubor sets in, the total period of time being about one minute longer than that necessary to establish a good red color. The limb is then placed in the horizontal position for about two to five minutes, during which time an electric heating pad is applied, care being taken to prevent the occurrence of a burn. The placing of the limb in these three successive positions constitutes a cycle, the duration of which is usually from six to ten minutes. These cycles are repeated over a period of about one hour, some six to seven cycles constituting a seance."

The Buerger boards as used at the Deaconess Hospital consist of two boards, each $\frac{3}{4}$ inch thick, 30 inches

[1]Buerger: Surgical Diagnosis and Treatment by American Authors, edited by A. J. Ochsner, Philadelphia, Lea & Febiger, *4*, 810, 1920.

long, and 11 inches wide, hinged at one end. In the middle of one board is a hinged tongue with a cleat on the other board so that the boards can be opened at an angle of 30°, 45° or 60° as desired. Patients may spend from three to six hours daily in doing these exercises.

2. Massage with lanolin or cocoa butter.

3. Not wear circular garters or sit with knees crossed.

4. If you have had or been threatened with gangrene, keep off the feet five or more minutes each hour of the day and if an amputation fifteen or more minutes. Protect the remaining leg by not getting fat. Preserve the feet or foot for ornament rather than for use.

Treatment of Abrasions of the Skin

1. Proper first-aid treatment is of the utmost importance even in apparently minor injuries. Consult a doctor immediately, especially if pain, redness, swelling or any inflammation is noticed.

2. Avoid irritating antiseptics. We do not use sulphonaphthol, lysol, creolin and similar coal tar disinfectants or iodine.

3. At once after injury some surgeons recommend applications of sterile gauze saturated with isopropyl alcohol or hexylresorcinol (S. T. 37). Keep wet for not more than thirty minutes by adding more of the antiseptic solution. Don't soak a sore foot.

4. Stay abed!

Common causes of gangrene are burns from a hot-water bag or electric heater (don't use such) and blisters due to ill-fitting shoes. If feet are cold, sleep in blankets or wear bed socks.

INFECTIONS OF THE SKIN

The skin of a diabetic should be kept exquisitely clean. A diabetic should be recognized for his clean skin and clean clothes. If his feet are kept as clean as his face, gangrene and infections will seldom occur. With patients over fifty years of age it is usually more important to look at their feet than their faces.

An infection makes the diabetes worse. When Case No. 3589 had a septic arm, 90 units of insulin failed to keep the urine sugar-free; when the infection was removed, sugar disappeared though the insulin was reduced to 30 units and carbohydrate and calories were increased. When Sister —— had an infected knee it was necessary to begin insulin and increase it to 45 units, but when recovery occurred, no insulin was required. It makes little difference whether the infection is general, as in pneumonia, or local, as in the case of a boil, a carbuncle, an abscessed tooth, an infected finger or toe, an inflamed tonsil, appendix or gall-bladder. Therefore, all infections should be promptly and energetically treated.

In the presence of an infection the diet is simplified and the substitutions employed as given on pages 67 and 191, Tables 5 and 11. Regular meals are replaced by more frequent feedings and therefore the dosage of insulin must be changed. In addition to the customary dose of insulin before breakfast one can add regular or crystalline as needed according to the accompanying schedule, every three, four or six hours according to the results of the Benedict test.

Red	Orange	Yellow	Green	Blue
16	12	8	4	0

A similar rule is often followed during surgical procedures (See page 55) and with surgical convalescents. As with most complications, strict control of the diabetes yields unexpectedly good results.

Itching

Pruritus pudendi (itching of the genitals) frequently occurs in diabetes and will usually vanish within a few days after the disappearance of sugar from the urine, but occasionally not until two weeks later. General pruritus, on the other hand, is exceptional, may be annoying and persist for weeks. It does not occur in young diabetics. If local pruritus does not clear up promptly, as the urine becomes sugar-free, an examination will probably disclose a prolapse, leukorrhea, urinary incontinence or a monilial infection. Rest in bed, absolute cleanliness, simple douches and the simplest of ointments are indicated. The free use of oil to prevent irritation during micturition is helpful. There may be cases where $\frac{1}{4}$ skin unit doses of Roentgen-ray become necessary to allay the itching. The salicylic and sulphur ointment, described in the next paragraph, occasionally gives good results. In some instances a physician may prescribe nupercaine ointment. Recently benadryl has been employed especially when there is an allergic cause. Obtundia ointment or Italian Balm is sometimes helpful. Use a fatty soap and temporarily bathe less often. Search for the cause. Be sure to ask for the help of a dermatologist or gynecologist if improvement is not prompt.

Epidermophytosis (Athlete's Foot)

Many people are affected with itching, scaling, cracking or blisters on the feet, especially between the toes. This condition is often a ringworm infection or epidermophytosis, as it is called, and is caused by a vegetable parasite which grows in the skin. It is less common now than formerly. It is particularly dangerous to diabetics, because it leads to scratching and by softening of the skin between the toes allows an entry to more dangerous infections. The disease is usually acquired by walking barefoot on the floors of shower baths, dressing and locker rooms, infected bath mats or any floor or floor covering where others who have it have walked in their bare feet.

The disease most commonly shows itself as a slight cracking or scaling, giving the appearance of dead, white skin between the fourth and fifth toes. The so-called soft corn is one form of this infection. The skin may look parboiled. In more severe cases groups of small deep blisters come on the soles of the feet and the palms of the hands. This form usually itches intensely. Most cases are worse during hot weather or when wearing shoes and stockings which heat the feet.

PREVENTION AND TREATMENT
OF ATHLETE'S FOOT

1. Wash the feet with soap and water daily.

2. Dry the feet with a paper towel or with a towel which will not be used on the rest of the body.

3. Stand on a clean bath mat, a newspaper or paper towel when you get out of the bath.

4. Never walk on any floors barefoot.

5. Do not wear wool stockings next to the skin— wear thin socks inside which can be boiled.

6. Do not wear shoes which heat the feet.

7. Use this dusting powder on feet, in shoes and bath slippers.

	Grams
Salicylic acid	2
Benzoic acid	2
Talc	100

8. With signs of the disease rub a little of this ointment every night on the affected parts.

	Grams
Salicylic acid	2
Precipitated sulphur	2
Petrolatum Jelly	30

9. Wash your hands after touching your feet.

10. Don't scratch if feet itch—put on ointment.

Certain of the angry eruptions seen about the genitals, buttocks, in the groins, armpits or under the breasts are likewise due to a similar infection. These usually yield promptly to treatment when the urine becomes sugar-free and the sugar in the blood falls. If they do not with scrupulous cleanliness, careful drying after bathing, dusting with a small quantity of a simple dusting powder see a skin specialist.

Boils

Today physicians will usually employ antibiotics in combating infections of the skin and the course of treatment is thereby greatly shortened; nevertheless, Dr. Bowen's[1] rules for cleanliness given in 1917 still hold.

If there is the slightest tendency to boils (furunculosis) at once adopt the simple measures which in part are here recorded. Take a shower bath twice a day with soap and water, using a fresh piece of sterilized gauze and powdered or liquified soap; dry the skin with a freshly boiled towel without rubbing or blot it with paper towels so as to avoid breaking open any pustule; the whole body is then bathed and dried with 70 per cent alcohol alone. "This procedure—thorough bathing and soaping, the application of 70 per cent alcohol is repeated, morning and night. A further point of vital importance relates to the clothing that is worn next to the skin. Every stitch of linen worn next to the skin should be changed daily, and in the case of extensive furunculosis all the bedclothing that touches the individual, as well as the nightclothing, should be subjected to a daily change."

[1] Bowen: Jour. Am. Med. Assn., *55*, 209, 1910; Boston Med. and Surg. Jour., *176*, 96, 1917.

"The washed neck, like the watched pot, never boils," my friend Dr. F. Gorham Brigham often told patients.

Carbuncles

Carbuncles are similar to boils, but more serious. They should be treated invariably by a surgeon from the start. Carbuncles are dreadfully dangerous of themselves and also because they make the diabetes so much worse. Fortunately now they are comparatively rare. Still more fortunately, with penicillin the dreadful mortality has been abolished and today operations in the majority of cases are avoided. *I remember the time when every other patient with a carbuncle died.* Prompt treatment today gives miraculous results. In fact we probably do not have more than one admission in 3000 for a carbuncle and the need of operation seldom exists. Today patients are much cleaner than formerly.

Poison Ivy

The best way to prevent poisoning from ivy is to know the appearance of the plant and keep strictly away from it. If you have touched it, however, washing over the skin exposed to the poison with a 5 per cent alcoholic solution of ferric chloride will entirely prevent an attack. If you cannot get this, use alcohol and follow it by a thorough scrubbing with laundry soap and water.

When the eruption has appeared it is too late to use these measures as preventives. Various antidotes are now available at a reliable pharmacy.

16

CONSTIPATION AND DIARRHEA

CONSTIPATION

THE bowels should move daily. If they do not, I think it generally means a poor bringing-up in childhood or gross neglect in later life. To this end nothing compares in effectiveness with the cultivation of regular habits and hours for this purpose. Time is required, and one-half hour, or even more, assigned to the toilet at the same time of the day for three successive days will often bring relief from constipation and this will persist for months. The coarse vegetables and fruits of the diet may prove quite sufficient, but it is essential to impress upon the patient the necessity of preparing coarse vegetables in a simple manner. It is perfectly possible to cook cabbage, cauliflower, turnips, parsnips, radishes, cucumbers and onions so as to be unirritating to the digestive tract and yet preserve their laxative qualities. This is important because the prolonged and careless use of coarse vegetables may bring on the spastic type of constipation which renders their abandonment for a period almost necessary. Caution should be exercised in the use of bran because temporary intestinal obstruction may result from its collection as a dry mass in the rectum and this necessitates its removal by hand. We have not given it at all for years. One or two glasses of water taken while dressing are helpful. Mineral oil used in place of olive oil, as an ingredient of mayonnaise salad dressing, is excellent, but it is not a good plan to use mineral oil month in and month out. It may remove fat-soluble vitamins. Mineral oil and milk of magnesia, each a tablespoonful more or less, is efficacious. Never purge the bowels, but depend upon an enema or upon simple laxatives, such as milk of magnesia; aloin, grain $\frac{1}{5}$; fluid extract of cascara sagrada, 10 to 30 drops; extract cascara sagrada, 5 grains. The ordinary compound rhubarb pill, although now less easily obtainable in any drug store, was the cathartic most in use at the Deaconess Hospital. These are very satisfactory. In certain rhubarb pills the presence of peppermint or salicylate may cause the excretion in the urine of an acid which can be confused with the diacetic acid of acid poisoning and thus lead to unwarranted alarm.

Citrate of magnesia in liquid form is contraindicated. In one preparation examined there was found 11 per cent of sugar. The amount of sugar in one bottle was more than 2 tablespoonfuls.

If the patient has not had a movement for several days, at the beginning of treatment give an enema and follow by some simple cathartic or mild laxative, and then give another enema twelve to twenty-four hours later; but do not purge the patient. Gain enough is obtained if a movement is produced once in twenty-four hours when it has only been taking place once in seventy-two. In other words, do not upset any patient who is in a tolerable state.

Case No. 559 warded off constipation by sawing wood, and Case No. 265 regulated his bowels by eating daily a slice of raw cabbage for breakfast. This is one of the reasons why cabbage next to lettuce is the most useful diabetic vegetable.

If blood is ever passed by the bowels, its source should be found and the cause eliminated. Don't be content with a diagnosis of hemorrhoids unless completely justified by examination. This generally means not only a digital examination, but inspecting the lower bowel with a proctoscope and usually an *x*-ray after a barium enema.

DIARRHEA

The reverse of constipation, diarrhea, is rare in diabetes, but occasionally is very troublesome and taxes the doctor's skill. Relief is obtained only by removal of the underlying cause. It is a serious complication. When it occurs the patient should go to bed immediately, keep warm and live upon hot water, broths, hot weak tea and strained oatmeal gruel which is thoroughly cooked and made with water. The half ounce, 15 grams, of dry oatmeal used for breakfast will make one-half pint of gruel. Temporarily being without food for a few hours is allowable, but this should not go on for long. The carbohydrate of the diet should be continued in the simplest form, such as gruels, crackers, toast, rice, macaroni or ginger ale. For their carbohydrate content see food tables, pages 287–296. Broths are most desirable because of their content of salt and they can be thickened with weighed (measured) quantities of flour or rice. A tablespoonful of flour weighs about 6 grams and is the equivalent of about 5 grams carbohydrate. See also Table 11, page 191, for the equivalent of the standard diet in simple and unirritating form.

The return to the diabetic diet is rendered easy by the use of cottage cheese, soft cream cheese, lean meats, oatmeal, milk, cream, biscuits, toast, eggs, puréed vegetables. The carefully prepared tender vegetables are frequently better borne than a diet containing considerable quantities of albuminous and fatty food. Milk should be boiled and taken with a teaspoon. Take liquids between rather than at meals.

If diarrhea exists, lime water could be employed or a portion of the allowed bread could be crumbled into the milk. Milk is also satisfactorily diluted with Vichy Célestin or Kalak Water. During infections orange juice (10 per cent carbohydrate) is desirable, but following abdominal operations ginger ale, which is about the same strength, is preferable, because it is less likely to cause cramps. I think surgeons should employ thickened strained soups and rice far more often than they do. It is easier, I know, to order intravenous glucose, but that is expensive.

TABLE 11.—A SUBSTITUTE FOR STANDARD DIET

Useful in the Treatment of Patients with Infections or Digestive Disturbances

Food	Carbo-hydrate, grams	Protein, grams	Fat, grams
Milk, 960 cc. (1 quart).........	48	32	32
20 per cent cream, 120 cc. ($\frac{1}{4}$ pint.	4	4	24
Bread, 90 grams (3 large slices)	45	8	0
Oatmeal, 30 grams dry (240 gms. cooked).....................	20	5	2
Egg, 1.......................	0	6	6
Butter, 30 grams.............	0	0	25
	117	55	89
	4	4	9
Total Calories................	468	220	801

Cottage cheese made of skimmed milk—30 to 60 grams—once or twice a day if more food is desirable.

If liquid is not retained by mouth it may be necessary to give salt solution and even 5 per cent glucose solution intravenously. If there is any suggestion of food remaining in the stomach this should be removed by lavage. The lower bowel should be cleared with an enema, and if even a trace of blood is noted, in addition to a routine digital examination of the rectum, the entire rectum should be explored with a proctoscope and an examination by x-ray. The physician may administer an opiate or he may give a teaspoonful of bismuth subcarbonate before each meal and after each loose movement. Rest in bed is the essential and the best sort of treatment. Diarrhea, especially diarrhea alternating with constipation, is a serious state and a doctor should be consulted. He will wish to exclude malignant disease, ulcerative colitis, or dysentery by examination of the rectum with a speculum and x-ray of the entire digestive tract.

Diarrhea may necessitate the decrease or the increase of insulin. As a result of the loose movements, the carbohydrate of the food is less well absorbed, and in consequence the insulin has less carbohydrate upon which to act and an insulin reaction may take place. On the other hand, with vomiting and diarrhea the body is forced to depend upon its own protein and fat for nourishment and may consume so much of these without any carbohydrate at the same time that acid poisoning takes place, and this can easily go on to coma. In the presence of acidosis insulin acts less efficiently and hence the demand for an increase in the dosage of insulin.

Upon all such occasions it is safer to reduce the protamine zinc insulin and supplement it with small and frequent doses of crystalline insulin. The same general rule can be followed as in the case of infections. (See page 183.)

Purgation and fasting were the weapons used by Guelpa to get his patients sugar-free, and they were most efficacious. Consequently, when these conditions occur by chance in a patient caution is demanded or else a little insulin will produce an unexpectedly great effect.

Diarrhea in any diabetic is dangerous. Call the doctor.

Nocturnal Diarrhea

Nocturnal diarrhea is a troublesome complaint and is especially annoying because the bowels are often incontinent. It occurs once or twice in a thousand cases. Such a complication requires careful investigation. This type of diarrhea is frequently associated with an absence of the normal hydrochloric acid in the gastric juice, possible deficiency of pancreatic secretion, and dependent upon an intestinal neuritis. Treatment is directed to offset these states. At times intramuscular injections

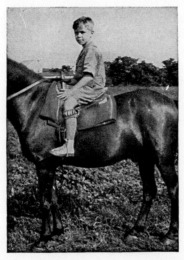

Fig. 24.—Case No. 2560 in August 1924; onset diabetes in 1921 at six years of age; in 1959 he is a hardworking lawyer, married with three children. When in law school he found it necessary to resume exercise.

of crude liver extract prove efficacious, but these must be continued for months. I do not recall having encountered an instance of nocturnal diarrhea in a patient whose diabetes was under control.

Caution.—Pain in the abdomen should never be neglected nor should delay in seeking medical advice for it be permitted. Even in health it may be difficult and require time to determine exactly the cause of abdominal pain. In a diabetic if a serious cause for the

13

pain is present acidosis may also develop within a few hours and obscure the signs and symptoms upon which the doctor must depend in making a diagnosis. The result may be confusion resulting in death. Do not give castor oil or other strong cathartics at such a time. They may cause an inflamed appendix to rupture. Let the doctor decide! Appendicitis is dreadfully serious. I was fortunate to have my appendix out at the age of 86. Ex-President Hoover according to the newspapers had his gall stones operated upon at the age of 83. From his example thousands of lives may be saved. An appendix or gall stones in a bottle by the side of a patient's bed does not cause worry.

17

SURGERY IN DIABETES

THE surgeon is the diabetic's friend. It is the surgeon who cures the infections which make his disease worse, extracts his bad teeth and poor tonsils, removes his appendix, takes out his gall stones or thyroid, thereby in some cases almost causing the diabetes to disappear, or hastens recovery from tuberculosis by an operation on his lung. Finally, it is the surgeon who often can relieve the diabetic from the suffering of gangrene by the amputation of his leg, or, better still, now save it by the removal of a toe or grafting in a new blood vessel and, best of all, cure a cancer by its early detection and excision. By the skill and cooperation of the surgeon's brothers, the ophthalmologists and obstetricians, blind diabetics often can recover their sight and mothers can have the joy of bearing a living child. Today over one-third of the quota of our hospital diabetic beds are occupied by diabetics with surgical complications, despite the fact that dreaded carbuncles, mastoid disease and lesser infections now are cured, without surgical intervention, by medical means with antibiotics and chemotherapy. Surgical mortality in diabetes has now been reduced to less than 3 per cent at the New England Deaconess Hospital.

Every other diabetic is operated upon during the course of his disease. Diabetics are just as liable to diseases requiring the surgeon's help as non-diabetics and, indeed, rather more so, because infections make the diabetes worse and it is imperative to get rid of them. Gall stones are common in diabetics and probably 25 per cent of those above thirty years of age have them. Gall stones precede rather than follow diabetes. Appendicitis occasionally occurs and is easily confused with diabetic coma, and more rarely with a reaction due to protamine zinc insulin. If the diagnosis is suggestive but uncertain, it is better to "take the trick" and get rid of it, and increasingly so the younger the individual. Diseased tonsils and abscessed teeth require removal. Carbuncles are serious, but if treated early the danger of death disappears. The most common surgical ailments are those of the lower extremities due to gangrene or chronic infections involving the bone. Such conditions begin unobtrusively in elderly people, because old peoples' feet are not sensitive and so injuries, whether from shoes or from burns, cause little pain, and an old man may walk around all day with a tack imbedded in the sole of his foot and not realize it. A fissure between the toes produced by epidermophytosis (athlete's foot) often is the source of inflammation which is responsible for weeks in a hospital. If neglected, these abrasions, cuts, cracks or burns of the skin become infected and the infection burrows deeply into the tissues and joints because the resistance is low, due to poor circulation. As a result amputation of a toe, foot or leg may be necessary. Picking, cutting, or tearing a callus or a corn, or pricking a blister may lead to such an infection. Corns on the upper side of the toes are especially dangerous, because so often these become infected and the joint in turn is involved. Take advantage of a chiropodist's skill. At the first sign of even a minor foot infection refer the patient immediately to a surgeon. Let him have the responsibility for further treatment.

If a diabetic washes his feet every night, he can discover trouble with the feet early, should it occur. Corns and calluses can be softened and rubbed off with gauze, pumice stone or emery boards. Do not prick a blister. Put that responsibility upon the surgeon. The majority of the surgical diabetic beds at the hospital are still filled with patients who have gangrene or infections of the feet, and these conditions are really to a very large extent needless. Fortunately, however, deaths from gangrene have dropped from 8 per cent to 1 per cent in our group.

Modern methods make the surgery upon diabetics safe and insulin allows any type of anesthesia which is necessary. See page 173. Should ether be employed, the liver is protected by the patient being operated upon early in the morning so that carbohydrate from the preceding evening meal will still be stored in it. If the operation is later in the day, it is safer to depend upon intravenous glucose in normal salt solution. Ginger ale, broths, water gruels and, except in the case of abdominal operations, orange juice can be employed soon after the operation. Doctor and surgeon, however, must work hand in hand to get the most successful results. It is wiser to operate when the urine is sugar-free, but it is wrong to put off an operation, even if not sugar-free, should the surgical condition be growing worse. Insulin is given according to the need and, as meals are irregular, more by the hour than by the day, depending upon the state of the patient and as described. (See page 55.) One tries to keep the urine sugar-free but is usually unsuccessful for a day or two following operation.

Often a patient wonders why a doctor, as well as a surgeon visits him twice daily, before and after an operation. The reasons are plain. It is essential to keep the diabetes well controlled, and the doctor has more experience and time to do this than the surgeon.

Years ago cancer was rare in diabetics and no wonder, because they died so young and lived so short a time. It is different today, because they live to be so old and three times as long. Indeed, 9 per cent of our cases die of cancer. But cancer we have proved bears no relation to diabetes. Especially watch for cancer in the digestive tract and lungs, where it is easily overlooked.

I think fewer diabetics should die of cancer than any other group of people in the world of similar age, because diabetics are under such close supervision of physicians that the cancer should be detected earlier and in a more operable stage.

Just as the diagnosis of diabetes in a child is made with the onset of coma similarly, in an adult, it is often first recognized with gangrene. Diligent search will disclose the disease has been burrowing unnoticed for years and has brought on profound degenerative changes in blood vessels. The supposedly mild or moderately severe surgical diabetic is really in a far more serious condition than the child, as Kendall Emerson, Jr., has emphasized, because of the prolonged pre-diabetic state.

18

DIABETIC COSTS

THE DIET of a diabetic patient with its fresh vegetables, fruit, milk, eggs and meat is somewhat expensive,
but it costs far less if the disease is controlled than if
uncontrolled. In the latter state the waste of food in
the form of calories lost as sugar in the urine is enormous.

The cost of treating the disease is small compared
with the cost of treatment of its complications, which is
huge. I doubt if a diabetic diet costs over one-quarter
more than the standard American diet. An attack of
diabetic coma involves, on the average, a minimum
expense of $100; a sore toe with spread of inflammation
into the entire foot or leg often $500 to $1,000; the
acquirement of tuberculosis $2500, or thereabouts in a
year. Diabetic doctors practically never develop coma,
seldom acquire gangrene and for years I have seen but
two diabetic doctors with tuberculosis. Lay diabetic
patients, too, should avoid these extravagant complications. Somebody pays for all of these, even if the patient does not. This is one of the reasons for building
the Hospital Teaching Clinic (See page 201) so that
patients at little expense can learn to avoid such costly,
serious and unnecessary complications. If they go
without cigarettes, much of the difference in cost is
saved.

Case No. 1171 told me that before treatment was
begun, he ate 13 eggs for breakfast, not by any means
as a stunt, but because he wanted them.

Case No. 1147, a lady, aged thirty-five years, ate a
dozen eggs a day, and in response to my request gave

(199)

me a report of her daily diet before she began treatment. This was estimated to contain carbohydrate 179 grams, protein 194 grams and fat 327 grams, but I suspect the carbohydrate must have been much greater before treatment actually commenced. Although the diet contained 60 calories per kilogram body weight instead of the normal 30 calories, the patient, while upon it, lost 66 pounds in a little over two and a half years. The reason for this was apparent, for on October 6, 1916, the volume of the urine was estimated at 6000 cc. (6 quarts) and the sugar was found to be 5 per cent, or 300 grams (10 ounces), the equivalent of a loss of 1200 calories in the urine in twenty-four hours, or about four-fifths of 1 pound of body weight. In one year the weight of sugar lost would amount to 240 pounds. The duration of her diabetes was 5.5 years; she died in September 1919 of diabetic coma, three years before insulin was available.

Case No. 295 voided in twenty-four hours, on October 23–24, 1909, approximately 10 quarts of urine (nearly 20 pounds), containing 680 grams of sugar, the equivalent of 2720 calories. The weight of his urine for one day was equal to one-fifth of that of his body. In other words, he lost in the urine 54 calories per kilogram, an amount sufficient in calories to supply almost double his own needs if taken in the form of food which he could assimilate.

Diabetic patients with acid poisoning lose calories in the urine in the form of ketone bodies (acetone, diacetic acid, β-oxybutyric acid) as well as of sugar. The quantity of acid bodies thus lost is quite considerable. These acid bodies represent wasted food just as much as does the sugar in the urine. Case No. 344 is a good illustration of this. On December 25–26, 1911, he excreted 188 grams of sugar, the equivalent of (188 $\times$ 4) 752 calories, and in addition 55 grams of acid bodies, equivalent to (55 $\times$ 5) 275 calories. Acid intoxication is really a dreadful robber, for besides stealing the food of a patient, it frequently steals his life! Against it the diabetic can insure himself by not overeating, particularly by not overeating of protein and fat, and by keeping the urine sugar-free with diet, exercise and insulin.

The diabetic can save money if discretion is employed. Oleomargarine or other preparations may be substituted for butter and employed instead of bacon and cream. Fat in the form of vegetable fat is much cheaper than animal fat and preferable. Vegetables, whether fresh or canned, can be purchased in bulk. Broth is expensive and a luxury. The home canning of vegetables in diabetic families should be encouraged. A garden is a great advantage but even 3 per cent vegetables must be consumed with discretion. A diabetic boy took a salt cellar with an ounce of salt into the tomato patch and ate 35 tomatoes one morning!

Lettuce may be the best vegetable for a diabetic, but cabbage is the cheapest. Patients seldom tire of cabbage any more than normal individuals tire of potato. Perhaps this is because it can be served in so many different forms. Fats are costly as compared with carbohydrate foods, but there is great variation in the cost of fat.

The total expense of treatment of diabetes, including all diabetics, has decreased markedly in the last decade, although for one diabetic for one day in a hospital it has risen. Teaching is cheaper than nursing and in the Hospital Teaching Clinic the duration of stay is halved and in fact, on March 2, 1959, was reduced one dollar a day per patient. We hope all hospitals soon will adjust their rates and make their charges according to the care required. Patients remain a few days instead of a few weeks. More and more are learning details of treatment in a doctor's office. The use of insulin allows more food in the form of carbohydrate and carbohydrate is

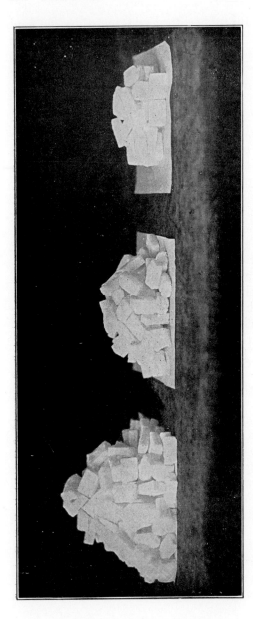

FIG 25.—Sugar, Measured as Lump Sugar, Lost in the Urine in One Day by Untreated Diabetic Patients.

Case No. 295
A Severe Diabetic
680 grams a day
546 pounds (1½ barrels) a year

Case No. 1147
A Moderate Diabetic
300 grams a day
240 pounds (⅔ barrel) a year

Case No. 653
A Mild Diabetic
174 grams a day
140 pounds (⅖ barrel) a year

The modern treatment of diabetes is so good that patients and their friends often forget how savage and serious diabetes really was and still can be if treatment is neglected.

cheaper than protein and fat. The cost of insulin dropped from 5 cents for one unit to about one cent for three units. Perhaps the most important factor of all is that relatively expenses have dropped, because patients are so much more vigorous that now they can be self-supporting.

Much more can be done in reducing expenses for diabetics. Hospital costs are shockingly high. They could be materially lowered if patients were classified according to nursing care required. Many are ambula-

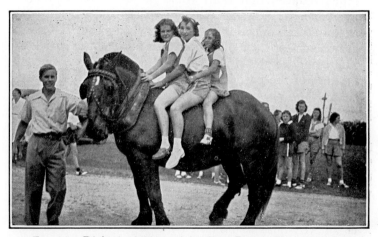

Fig. 26.—Diabetic children of the Clara Barton Birthplace Camp spend every other Sunday afternoon in the summer on our farm. Recently, in 1958, there were 82. It was quite an undertaking to give each one a horseback ride until the problem was solved by Peggy, who loved to carry three at a time

Don't you think our technician, Peggy, also prefers to do three blood sugars in one batch rather than each one of the three separately? Even Mollie says it is easier to bake three loaves of bread in the oven at one time on one day than to heat up the oven for a single loaf three times.

Have a heart! Don't ask for an immediate report of a blood sugar except in emergencies. Arrange for tests on a wholesale basis and reduce laboratory work for the technician and she will reduce costs. Try to get the Laboratory to sell you 10 blood sugar tests in a year at a wholesale rate.

tory and could go to a dining room or cafeteria. By light housework the patients benefit from the exercise, and incidentally lower costs. (See Hospital Teaching Clinic, page 201.) Nurses aides could often replace nurses. Fees for laboratory tests could be greatly lowered if done on a wholesale basis and reports on the spot not demanded. It requires nearly as much time to perform one blood sugar test as ten tests. By arranging for the performance of these tests wholesale for a group of doctors or patients, the outlay would be so much reduced that they would be far more generally available. The same policy applies to roentgen-ray examinations of the chest which now, on a routine basis, are one dollar for a photoroentgen film. Class instruction could be greatly extended and should include the families of the patients. Try to help not only the patients, but also to urge them to try to prevent the disease in their relatives by telling them not to be fat.

The reason I like to treat diabetics is that once in a while I think I can do them some good and I confess I enjoy telling them of some experience with a former patient which might be of use. Another reason is that diabetics, like most people, have all kinds of troubles, and I take for granted that diabetes is not the whole story and then try to find out what else is the matter. Finally, I believe routine health examinations are desirable and that if a diabetic comes to a doctor every three months there will be a good chance of picking up some serious disease in so early a stage that it can be cured and thus, because of the diabetes, a life will be saved, which without diabetes might be lost.

I never forget one patient who was so fortunate as to tumble downstairs and break her collarbone. I saw her for that and incidentally discovered a cancer of the breast which quite likely she might not have told me about; and twenty years later at the age of eighty-four she succumbed to a totally different disease without any recurrence of the cancer. When a doctor sees a faithful patient regularly and misses a diagnosis, that breaks his heart. Perhaps it is to ease my medical conscience for worse medical sins that I pay patients three dollars on the spot when I miss their veins in taking blood for a blood sugar test. Moreover, when I can't hit a vein, it will be an indication that it is time to look for another job somewhere else.

19

EXPECTATION OF LIFE—PROGNOSIS

"Grow old along with me!
The best is yet to be,
The last of life, for which the first was made:
Our times are in His hand
Who saith 'A whole I planned,
Youth shows but half; trust God; see all nor be afraid!'"

Browning: Rabbi Ben Ezra

A NATURAL measure of longevity is the average length of life, or, as it is also often called, the expectation of life at birth. It tells us the age in years to which, on the average, a newborn baby will survive. In 1900 it was about 49 years—48.2 years for white males and 51.1 for white females; in 1955 it was 69.6 years—67.3 for white males and 73.7 for white females. Similarly, the expectation of life at any other age as, for example, age thirty, tells us how many more years, on the average, a person of thirty years of age can expect to live.

As the individual grows older his expectation of life naturally diminishes. This will be seen in Table 13, which exhibits the expectation of life at successive ages of the white male and white female population of the United States in 1949–1951, as prepared in the Satistical Bureau of the Metropolitan Life Insurance Company.

How long can a diabetic live? That depends largely on his common sense. He may live to a ripe age, but will he do so? Today his expectancy is about three-fourths as long as that of a non-diabetic. The question cannot be answered satisfactorily for many, many years, because the discovery and use of insulin did not begin until 1922, and insulin was not generally employed until 1924. The course of the disease in children, more than anything else, throws light on the question.

Only 1.8 per cent of the diabetics I had seen up to 1914 survived twenty years, but this has increased to 42 per cent for 1956–1957, and in fact all with onset under forty years had lived an average of twenty or more years at this period. To show how rapidly the number of long duration cases is growing, particularly with children, I find that in 1934 the Joslin Clinic had 15 diabetics with onset in childhood of fifteen years' duration, but in November, 1952, of the 3246 children, 825 had had diabetes twenty years, 98 for thirty years and 5 for thirty-five years, but none for forty years. By 1957, out of a total of 4219 children with onset under 15 years of age, there were approximately 3351 cases known to be alive (80 per cent). Of this number 8 have lived over 40 years; 76 over 35 years; 215 over 30 years; 399 over 25 years and 917 over 20 years.

Many of my diabetics live longer after they have acquired diabetes than the average individual of similar age would be expected to live. The number I estimate at about 3000. And to such through the kindness of a friend I am able to give the medal, designed by Amelia Peabody, shown on page 210 of this book. The inscriptions upon it speak for themselves. The medal is made of bronze, but if the patient should live one-half again as long as his expectancy we would award a medal of silver and if so fortunate as to live twice as long as his expectancy, we formerly gave a medal of gold, but now the number is advancing so rapidly I fear it will be too much for our diabetes funds.

The longer life for diabetics has been summarized in a Bulletin published by the Statistical Department of the Metropolitan Life Insurance Company.[1] The death rates for all ages of life decreases uniformly and without

[1]Metropolitan Life Insurance Co. Statistical Bulletin, *38*, No. 1, 1958, Jan.

a single break from the earliest period 1898–1914
through that of the last, 1939–1945. With onset under
ten years the mortality has fallen 99 per cent and even
at age sixty it has decreased 72 per cent. This table of
death rates shows no halting tendency. Progress has
been uninterrupted. Evidently for diabetics all the
traffic lights are green.

PROPORTION OF FATAL CASES SURVIVING 20 YEARS OR LONGER

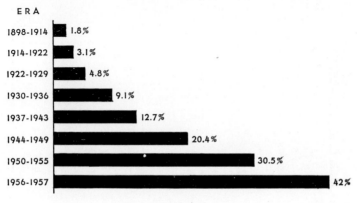

FIG. 27

Expectation of life in tabular form is shown in Table
14. This table, however, makes no allowance for improvements which may take place in the treatment of
diabetes in the coming generation and, therefore, under-
states rather than overstates the life expectancy of the
diabetic. As a matter of fact, it is a fair statement to
say that whatever the age of a diabetic at the onset of
his disease, his expectancy is approximately three-
fourths that of those of the same age about him without
allowance for new discoveries.

Are you just an average diabetic or are you above the
average in intelligence, backbone and courage? I hope
you belong to the latter class.

TABLE 12.—DURATION OF LIFE SUBSEQUENT TO ONSET OF DIABETES AMONG 18,055 DECEASED DIABETIC PATIENTS IN EACH OF THE IMPORTANT ERAS OF TREATMENT

(Number and Per Cent of Cases Classified According to Duration)
(Experience of Joslin Clinic, 1897–1957*)[1]

| Age Groups at Onset | Naunyn Era 1897–5/31/14 Duration Years | Allen Era 6/1/14–8/6/22 Duration Years | Banting Era | |
			8/7/22–12/31/29 Duration Years	1/1/30–12/31/36 Duration Years
All Ages	4.9†	6.1†	8.0†	10.3†
0–9	1.3	2.9	2.8	7.3
10–19	2.7	2.7	3.4	7.4
20–39	4.3	4.9	8.9	14.4
40–59	7.0	8.0	9.5	11.6
60 and over	4.4	6.4	5.5	7.0
Unknown	—	—	—	—

| Age Groups at Onset | Hagedorn Era | | Charles H. Best Era | |
	1/1/37–12/31/43 Duration Years	1/1/44–12/31/49 Duration Years	1/1/50–12/31/55 Duration Years	1/1/56–12/11/57 Duration Years
All Ages	12.1†	13.7†	15.6†	18.2†
0–9	10.3	18.5	20.6	26.4
10–19	11.4	16.2	20.1	23.5
20–39	16.9	18.8	21.8	25.1
40–59	13.4	14.9	16.2	18.7
60 and over	8.6	9.2	10.0	10.2
Unknown	—	—	—	—

*Deaths reported through December 11, 1957.
†Based on cases with known duration.
[1]Prepared by Statistical Bureau of Metropolitan Life Insurance Company.

TABLE 13.—EXPECTATION OF LIFE IN YEARS FOR UNITED STATES
1949—1951*

Age	Males White	Females White	Age	Males White	Females White
0	66.31	72.03	55	19.11	22.58
1	67.41	72.77	56	18.41	21.77
2	66.55	71.90	57	17.72	20.97
3	65.64	70.98	58	17.05	20.18
4	64.71	70.04	59	16.40	19.41
5	63.77	69.09	60	15.76	18.64
6	62.82	68.13	61	15.13	17.89
7	61.87	67.17	62	14.51	17.15
8	60.90	66.20	63	13.91	16.42
9	59.95	65.23	64	13.33	15.70
10	58.98	64.26	65	12.75	15.00
11	58.02	63.28	66	12.19	14.30
12	57.05	62.31	67	11.64	13.62
13	56.09	61.33	68	11.10	12.96
14	55.14	60.36	69	10.58	12.31
15	54.18	59.39	70	10.07	11.68
16	53.24	58.42	71	9.58	11.08
17	52.30	57.45	72	9.10	10.49
18	51.37	56.49	73	8.64	9.93
19	50.45	55.53	74	8.20	9.39
20	49.52	54.56	75	7.77	8.87
21	48.60	53.60	76	7.36	8.38
22	47.68	52.65	77	6.96	7.90
23	46.77	51.69	78	6.59	7.44
24	45.85	50.73	79	6.23	7.01
25	44.93	49.77	80	5.88	6.59
26	44.00	48.82	81	5.54	6.20
27	43.08	47.86	82	5.22	5.83
28	42.15	46.91	83	4.91	5.48
29	41.22	45.95	84	4.62	5.14
30	40.29	45.00	85	4.35	4.83
31	39.36	44.05	86	4.10	4.53
32	38.44	43.11	87	3.87	4.25
33	37.51	42.16	88	3.66	3.99
34	36.59	41.22	89	3.46	3.74
35	35.68	40.28	90	3.27	3.51
36	34.76	39.35	91	3.09	3.29
37	33.86	38.41	92	2.93	3.09
38	32.95	37.48	93	2.77	2.90
39	32.06	36.56	94	2.62	2.72
40	31.17	35.64	95	2.48	2.56
41	30.29	34.73	96	2.35	2.41
42	29.42	33.82	97	2.23	2.27
43	28.56	32.91	98	2.12	2.15
44	27.71	32.01	99	2.01	2.03
45	26.87	31.12	100	1.92	1.92
46	26.04	30.24	101	1.83	1.83
47	25.22	29.36	102	1.74	1.74
48	24.41	28.49	103	1.67	1.66
49	23.61	27.62	104	1.59	1.59
50	22.83	26.76	105	1.53	1.53
51	22.06	25.91	106	1.46	1.46
52	21.30	25.07	107	1.40	1.40
53	20.55	24.23	108	1.34	1.34
54	19.82	23.40			

*Compiled from: U.S. Vital Statistics-Special Reports, Tables 5 and 6, Vol. 41, No. 1, November 23, 1954.

14

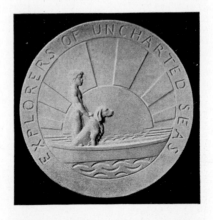

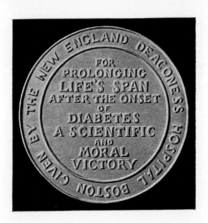

Fig. 28

To Those Individuals Who Have Conquered
Diabetes by Living Longer with It
Than They Were Expected to Live without It

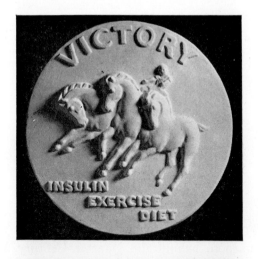

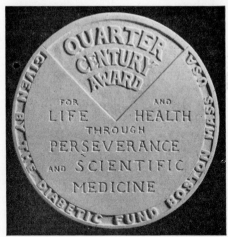

F<small>IG</small>. 29

T<small>HE</small> Q<small>UARTER</small> C<small>ENTURY</small> V<small>ICTORY</small> M<small>EDAL</small> <small>FOR</small> H<small>EALTH</small>

(*See page 212.*)

TABLE 14.—EXPECTATION OF LIFE

For White Persons in the General Population and for Diabetics
of the Joslin Clinic (1947–1951)

Age	United States 1949–1951	Diabetics 1947–1951
10	58.9	44.2
20	49.6	36.1
30	40.5	29.5
40	31.6	22.4
50	23.3	16.0
60	16.0	10.8
70	10.1	7.1

Quarter Century Victory Medal Diabetics

The purpose behind the Quarter Century Victory
Medal for diabetics was and is to spread the idea that
diabetics can live long and healthfully, to grant distinc-
tion to those who deserve it and to disclose what manner
of life and treatment has made this possible. The medal
was designed by Amelia Peabody in 1947 for The Diabetic Fund of the Boston Safe Deposit and Trust
Company and is awarded upon recommendation of its
Advisory Committee. To date 85 such medals have
been distributed and now in 1959, the average duration
of diabetes of the medalists is 33 years. The group is
remarkable in that on the whole it is symptomless. It
shows that diabetics can be in healthy condition 25
years after onset and it discloses that the reason is the
active, energetic treatment, particularly at the onset
of the disease. The recipients are explorers, discoverers.
They have demonstrated that not only have they lived,
but have lived more abundantly.

The conditions upon which the medal is granted are:

1. Proof that diabetes is of twenty-five years' duration.

2. Certification that the patient's condition is excellent on physical examination and on examination of the urine.

3. Certification by an accredited ophthalmologist that the eyes are free from complications.

4. Certification by an accredited roentgenologist that there is no evidence of calcification in the arteries.

X-Ray Films Needed:

Chest—PA and Lateral films taken at 6 ft. *Lumbar Spine*—Lateral film to show abdominal aorta. Bone technique—moderate density. *Pelvis*—AP view. Bone technique—moderate density. *Legs*—Lateral films of both legs. Films must extend 17 inches in the axis of the legs from (and including) the popliteal space to the ankle. Technique suggested for a patient of average size: 100 MA, 1 second, 58 KV at 40 inches with cardboard folders. *Ankles*—Lateral films of both ankles extending to a point below the os calcis and using cardboard folders.

We ask that the *x*-ray films be submitted to us to be looked over by the roentgenologists here who to date, with two exceptions, have passed on our 85 cases.

Applications should be submitted to:

Dr. Elliott P. Joslin, Chairman Advisory Committee
15 Joslin Road, Boston 15, Massachusetts

20

THE PREVENTION OF DIABETES

TRY to prevent the development of diabetes, but even if you do acquire it, discover it early and thus halt its progress.

It has been shown that in a dog with pancreas partially removed, experimental diabetes can be prevented if the dog is not overfed, and in a similarly prepared cat, made diabetic with injections of anterior pituitary extract, it can be cured if the blood sugar is kept normal. The amount of islet tissue which makes insulin in the pancreas may be substantially increased in an animal by treatment with anterior pituitary extract and this approach has been applied with some success in the alloxan diabetes of rabbits. The knowledge already gained is encouraging and eventually may be applicable to man. Whether success is attained in months or years, it is a satisfaction that these recent developments support the vigorous and aggressive measures thus far advocated to control the disease. Fight it from start to finish and victory is nearer now than ever before.

Heredity

It takes two to make a diabetic. See Chapters 21 and 22.

Obesity and the Diabetic

Since you cannot pick your parents and grandparents and thus avoid diabetes, do the next best thing and not get fat. According to the Northwestern National Life Insurance Company if a person is 10 pounds overweight, the average chances of death are increased 8 per cent; if 30 pounds overweight, 28 per cent; if 50 pounds overweight, 56 per cent; if 80 pounds overweight, 116 per cent. To be a few pounds overweight is all right until you are thirty-five years of age, but after that it is not allowable if there is any tendency to diabetes in your family, and indeed it is contrary to future good health under any circumstances. To inherit diabetes is blameless, but to acquire it through obesity when you have an hereditary tendency to it is blamable.

TABLE 15.—VARIATION FROM NORMAL OF MAXIMUM WEIGHTS AT OR PRIOR TO ONSET OF 1000 CASES OF TRUE DIABETES, CALCULATED FOR HEIGHT, AGE AND SEX. SECOND SERIES, 1926.

Age, years	*No. of cases*	*No. underweight*	*No. overweight*	*No. of normal weight*
0–10.......	43	19	8	16
11–20.......	84	24	27	33
21–30.......	112	11	80	21
31–40.......	172	8	153	11
41–50.......	244	7	207	30
51–60.......	252	2	220	30
61–70.......	79	5	66	8
71–80.......	14	1	11	2
1–80.......	1000	77	772	151

Diabetics in middle life are proverbially fat before the disease begins. Formerly, but now less commonly, it was often possible in a diabetic class of 30 persons to pick out 10 whose combined weights before the onset of the disease equalled one ton. The average weight of 1326 married diabetic women above the age of forty-five years coming to me for treatment was 181 pounds and of 111 single women 161 pounds. One must prevent overweight in married women. In a

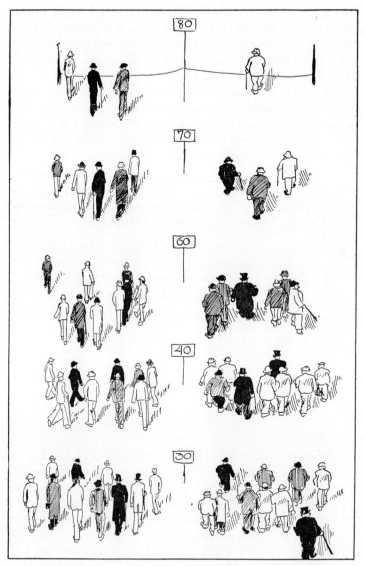

FIG. 30.—How 10 fat and 10 lean men fare as they walk
through life.

group of 1000 diabetics arranged by decade of onset there were only 77 who were underweight, 151 of standard weight but there were 772 who were overweight. It is most exceptional for a thin individual over forty years of age to get diabetes.

In middle life diabetes is overwhelmingly more common in women than in men and obesity is an important factor. I suspect it accounts in large measure for the predominance of diabetes in Jewish adults and in Negro women. Compare the weights of these two groups now with similar groups even a decade ago. It is especially notable that colored girls are now seldom overweight. Consequently, efforts for prevention should be concentrated upon women, and especially Jewish and Negro women. One must insist that these susceptible individuals do not get fat, particularly if there is also present an hereditary tendency to diabetes.

If one regards diabetes as a penalty of obesity, the greater the obesity the more likely is Nature to enforce it. A fat man generally has a fat wife, so it is not uncommon to encounter the disease in both heads of the family. Fat parents bring up fat children, so it is no wonder that diabetes is found in fat families. A fat nurse cuts a fat slice of bread and a thin nurse automatically cuts a thin slice. Obesity is so common in the Hebrew race that it is easy to understand that Dr. Hyman Morrison in 1916 found diabetes two and a half times more frequent in the Jewish population of Boston than among the rest of the inhabitants. Not many years ago I found that I had examined only one adult Jewish male and only one adult Jewish female who were underweight prior to the onset of their diabetes. The statistics of Israel should be of great value. Will the incidence of diabetes grow less?

Lack of exercise leads to overweight and thus is an indirect cause of diabetes. Disuse of the muscles, however, is also a direct factor, for it is largely in the

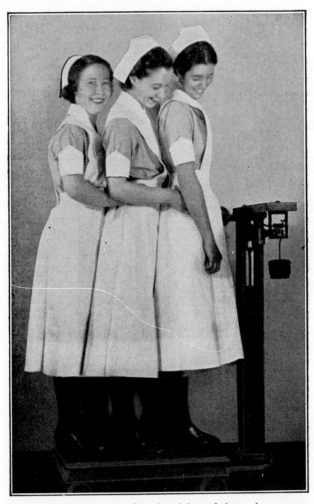

Fig. 31.—It took the combined weights of these three nurses to equal the weight—315 pounds—of one of my diabetic patients, case 4236. She lived 18 years with diabetes. I am happy to add that the three nurses in 1959 are alive and weigh 356 pounds.

muscles that the sugar formed from the food is consumed. The man who gives up an active outdoor life and is promoted to an office chair by this change becomes a promising candidate for diabetes. Policemen, firemen, aviators—beware! Very likely this is the reason diabetes is more often met with in those living in the city than in the country, because in the city there is less physical work. So, too, in a larger sense this may account to some degree for the increase in diabetes in recent years, because now we depend so much upon mechanical devices instead of our own muscles. Electricity and the automobile in the hereditarily predisposed are undoubtedly responsible for many cases of diabetes. Exercise is important in treatment of diabetes, but just as important in prevention.

An existing diabetes grows worse in the presence of any infectious disease, whether general like pneumonia, or local like tonsillitis or a boil; but it is yet to be demonstrated that an infection causes diabetes, save when it occurs in the region of the pancreas and gall bladder and there is even doubt about that. Neither an infection nor an injury makes diabetes permanently more severe.

Convalescence from Disease or Injury

Following an infection rapid gains in weight often occur during convalescence. I remember I gained 17 pounds in 17 days following my first attack of pneumonia in 1906 and then called a halt to overeating.

Pregnancy

During pregnancy sugar is apt to occur in the urine. Mild cases of glycosuria which go untreated in pregnancy may later in the same or in subsequent pregnancies become aggravated cases of diabetes. Particularly in families with a diabetic heredity when pregnancy occurs one should avoid overweight, test even more frequently for the presence of sugar and by glucose tolerance tests seek to disclose it early. Confinements should be followed by examinations of the urine every three months for a year, and thereafter every six months for life.

The gain in weight which so often follows cessation of nursing should be avoided. Mothers should not continue to eat for two persons when they stop feeding one. Gain in weight at the menopause is proverbial. *Fair, Fat* and *Forty*.

It has been said by Professor Hoet of Louvain that 90 per cent of the women whose infant weighed 5000 grams and 100 per cent of those weighing 6 kilograms will eventually develop diabetes. In 1901, a baby was born weighing $12\frac{1}{2}$ pounds. In 1926, the mother, and in 1947, the baby itself developed diabetes. The subsequent three children in the family, through the commonsense of the mother, were not fat children and thus far, 1959, have not developed the disease.

Gall Stones

Gall stones are about twice as common among diabetics over twenty-five years of age as among a similar group in the community at large. As gall stones are proverbially more frequent among women, it is of especial interest that females are now showing a higher incidence of diabetes than men. Gall stones often precede diabetes and may precipitate it by direct extension of infection to the head of the pancreas. This seems possible, because there the islands of Langerhans are few and the gall stone type of diabetes is mild, but I confess statistics do not support this idea.

My advice to non-diabetic patients with gall stones is to be operated upon not only because of the danger of repeated attacks of gall stones and of the danger of a subsequent cancer, but also because of the danger of the development of diabetes. To diabetic patients my advice is to have the gall stones removed when the conditions of time, place, surgeon, and physician are all propitious.

Illustrative Cases

Overweight predisposes to diabetes and I certainly know it. For the prevention of more than one-half of the cases of diabetes in this country no radical under-nutrition is necessary; the individual is simply asked to maintain the weight of his average fellowman. It is desirable to spread the information that those live longest who, above the age of thirty-five years, are 5 to 10 per cent below the average normal weight. Patients should be cautioned against gaining weight particularly after infectious diseases, during and after pregnancy, after operations for gall stones, and when changing from an active to a sedentary mode of life. Although emphasis is usually laid upon the appearance of sugar in the urine with a patient losing weight, it cannot be too strongly emphasized that it is a common occurrence for sugar to appear in the urine when a patient is gaining weight. The first hint of diabetes occurred in Case 1207 when she weighed 142 pounds in 1895, but the disease did not become established in full force until 1912, when her weight was 248 pounds.

The slow onset of diabetes is favorable for the prevention of the disease. There is good reason to believe that the outbreak can be postponed or even prevented. In children diabetes usually comes on more rapidly, but even in children this halting onset is occasionally seen and often a considerable interval occurs before the disease becomes permanent. Case 129 showed sugar in the urine in 1901, at the age of three years, her father wrote, "at a time when she appeared out of condition. Examining her frequently after that I failed to find it and did not look for it again until in February, 1905, when she appeared like a full-fledged case of diabetes."

Who would say that the onset of diabetes in George M., Case 2151, aged twenty years in 1912, could not have been prevented? His grandfather and father had diabetes. His weight was 29 per cent above standard for his age, and he reported eating two whole pies a day and a whole bottle of cream on his pudding on Sunday. He died in 1945 of high blood pressure and cirrhosis of the liver.

Combat the slightest hint of diabetes. Of 1900 patients who showed a mere trace of sugar but not enough to diagnose frank diabetes, Dr. Marble found that some 10 per cent later developed the disease. They were the cases with marked heredity, overweight or of Jewish ancestry. May we not have protected the remaining 90 from developing the disease by having cautioned them against overweight and overeating and by having urged them to exercise and lead hygienic lives and by urging them to test the urine frequently and to diet at the slightest presence of sugar.

Louisa Drumm. March 30, 1920, there came to my office a woman with diabetes. She was given the usual examination with suggestions for treatment, and as it was impractical for her to enter the hospital she was taught on the spot to examine her urine. She went home and shortly after contracted pneumonia and died. But in the intervening days amid her household cares she found time and took enough interest to examine the urine of 10 others in her boardinghouse, and in so doing discovered the presence of diabetes in a boy. She gave him sound advice and sent him to his own physician, who also subsequently died, and later the boy came to me with this story. On the day she learned the Benedict test and made these 10 urinary examinations for her friends, Louisa Drumm was aged seventy-nine years and four months. Can one not appropriately say to younger diabetic patients, "Go thou and do likewise?"

In Paris in 1955, Professor Raoul Boulin established a clinic for the "Prevention of Diabetes," especially among the hereditarily predisposed, those overweight and pregnant women. He took this step because he felt diabetes was not always irreversible and that one should cease saying:—"*Le médecin arrive trop tard.*" (The doctor arrived too late.) Among 364 cases predisposed to diabetes he found 52 true cases and 98 borderline cases. By early treatment of these latter he hoped to prevent the full development of diabetes.

21

HEREDITY

DIABETES is hereditary, but it takes two to make a diabetic. In other words, diabetes must be present in both parents or their ancestors. Suppose two diabetics should marry and have 100 children. Theoretically all these children should develop diabetes, but practically it has been calculated that only about 44 would acquire it, because the rest would succumb to other causes before they reached the age at which their diabetes would break loose. But even this statement is not quite so bad as it sounds. The chances are overwhelming that none of the children at birth would have diabetes. Among over 52,000 diabetics or individuals with sugar in the urine, I have not seen one congenital case and only 20 with onset in the first year of life. Only about one-third of the above 44 destined to have diabetes would get it under 40 years of age, another third between 40 and 55, and the remainder between the ages of 55 and 100 years. Estimates as above stated are being constantly revised.

It is the tendency to diabetes and not the actual disease which is inherited. Dr. Umber of Berlin tells the story of a child who entered the hospital with diabetes; ten years later the mother was admitted for the same cause; and again in ten years the grandmother came for treatment also with diabetes. Before the discovery of insulin diabetic children lived so short a time that we heard little about heredity, but in 1953 Dr. Priscilla White told me that among 800 of our cases who developed diabetes in childhood and had survived twenty or more years, there were 60 per cent who had relatives with the disease and I personally found 60 in a hundred successive cases whom I questioned in 1958, and presumably other cases would appear later. Among the relatives of a group of diabetic patients, Dr. White found that diabetes was seven times as common as among non-relatives, and in Florida the United States Public Health Service found it five times as common. Of course we are constantly finding new cases among the group and if we knew all the facts, undoubtedly it would be shown that every diabetic had a diabetic relative, unless the ancestors died so young that it had not appeared. Proof of the importance of heredity is steadily increasing.

Table 16, below, also illustrates forcibly the influence of heredity as a cause of diabetes.

TABLE 16.—A COMPARISON OF THE INCIDENCE OF DIABETES IN THE SIBLINGS (BROTHERS AND SISTERS) OF NON-DIABETICS, DIABETICS, DISSIMILAR AND SIMILAR TWINS, AND OF DIABETES IN THEIR PARENTS.

Type of population	Siblings, number	Per cent diabetic
Control................	862	0.6
Diabetic...............	2835	5.0
Dissimilar twin.........	29	7.0
Similar twin...........	19	63.0

When a diabetic marries a non-diabetic but one whose father or mother and sometimes brother or sister has diabetes, one-half of the children theoretically should develop the disease, but practically less than one-fourth. If two non-diabetics, but each of a diabetic family and thus carriers of the disease, marry, the ratio of the off-spring destined to diabetes theoretically would be 1 in 4, but again practically less than 1 in 8. But if a diabetic will choose a non-diabetic of a non-diabetic family

15

for a partner, none of the children should come down with the disease. Be careful then diabetics, with whom you fall in love. Remember, only 1 person in 3 in the United States has a diabetic relative, so that there are more than 120,000,000 available with a non-diabetic heredity for husbands or wives.

Diabetes unquestionably is a disease of the family. One must focus on the family to prevent it. Diabetic parents and grandparents should strive not only to care for themselves, but should endeavor to protect their posterity. Further, I think they should contribute to the study and care of other diabetics, so that if their descendants do develop the disease, treatment will be better than at present. Diabetics are bright and there are enough of them to care for one another. "Diabetes for the Diabetics" is a good slogan. Emphasize the prevention of obesity and the early detection of diabetes.

How can diabetes be prevented if there is a family tendency to it? Above all things do not become forty and fat, and if you are a diabetic put this same rule in force among your relatives and teach your descendants to avoid obesity. By this means much of the element of heredity probably can be overcome or postponed. Encourage the children to eat vegetables freely and fruits instead of ice-cream, sherbets and pastry desserts. Don't put them on a diabetic diet. Discourage candy or pure sugar as in ginger ale or similar sweet drinks. At any rate, seek to discover the disease early and make it a family custom to have the urine of each member examined on his or her birthday.

What is the effect of diabetes upon a race? We do not need to look far. In Jews the incidence may be two times as great as in Gentiles. Has it injured or helped the Hebrew race? Here is an experiment on a 12,000,000 scale. Suppose we watch it. Today the Jews are beginning to learn that they should not be so fat. In consequence I wonder what the incidence of diabetes will be in Jews in the next decades. I suspect that intermarriage between cousins will occur less frequently among Jews in the future than formerly.

In any crusade against diabetics marrying and having children, no consideration appears to have been given to possible advances in the treatment or prevention of the disease. Even a generation ago it was clear that progress in diabetes was imminent. And what of today with the almost complete abolition of diabetic coma, the diminishing death rate in the young, the relative safety in operations, through the use of sulfa drugs and antibiotics, all of which have followed the discovery of insulin. Yet all of these past achievements seem insignificant when one realizes the better scientific tools, the wider distribution of laboratories, and the greatly increased number of really skilled research workers, all now available for a successful attack on the disease.

The actual number of individuals with a diabetic heredity is huge. Over and over again in various parts of the world when talking before mixed audiences I have polled those present and found that about one in five had a diabetic relative. Recently among 68 nurses in training at the New England Deaconess Hospital 35 per cent reported diabetes in their families. This high incidence is true, although few of us know of what our grandparents, not to say our great-grandparents, have died and much less our great-great-grandparents. Few are as sure that their great-great-great-great-great-grandfather did not die of diabetes as I am that mine did not, because it is recorded that he, John Proctor, was hung on Gallows Hill in Salem in 1692. Fortunately for my family, and me, my great-great-great-great-great grandmother, who was to have shared his fate, was spared because she was pregnant, and before her child was born the English Government had put an end to the Salem witchcraft orgy.

If diabetes is hereditary, one asks, why not end it by

limiting the progeny of diabetics? From what has been said, I believe that is plainly impracticable. We know that there are in the United States at the present time about 2,000,000 diabetics and at least one-half as many more individuals in whom the disease is not recognized. These have so many relatives who carry the trait of diabetes that such a number could not be sterilized. To attempt to eliminate diabetes in this way, furthermore, is impossible because in most cases one cannot know who is to become diabetic. I have two families in whom one of the parents has diabetes and has had fourteen children, of whom twelve are living, and in the other family the father has diabetes and there are fifteen living children.

To lessen the number of future diabetics, first, one diabetic should not marry another diabetic and preferably not into a family in which diabetes is common. Second, all relatives of diabetics should remember that they are at least five times as liable to develop the disease as those in non-diabetic families, and therefore should be on the watch for it. Third, especially the relatives of diabetics should avoid overeating, because at least 85 per cent of diabetics from middle life on are fat before the diabetes appears and by avoiding obesity they may escape the disease.

Our data on heredity show very few instances involving 5 or even 4 generations. New light upon heredity will surely be disclosed in the next few years.

22

THE MARRIAGE OF DIABETICS

SHOULD a diabetic marry? Yes or no.

If marriage is contemplated by a diabetic, his or her future partner and both families should know the facts. Diabetes can be controlled and diabetics can marry, live happily for years and years and have healthy non-diabetic children, but this is only 100 per cent true when the diabetes is controlled and there is diabetes in only one of the contracting parties. Manifestly, as in the case of non-diabetics, both individuals before entering upon matrimony should furnish a doctor's certificate not only of a healthy body, but in addition the diabetic individual should furnish evidence as to whether the diabetes is controlled. The non-diabetic girl, or even boy, might well ask: (1) has the diabetic been accepted for insurance? (2) has the diabetic financial support? and (3) if holding a job, does the employer know of the existence of diabetes?

The contracting parties should have been acquainted with each other long enough to realize what the treatment of diabetes by diet, insulin, exercise and pills involves.

A diabetic should not marry another diabetic and have children. It is inadvisable for a diabetic to marry into a family with a marked diabetic heredity. See Chapter 21, page 228.

Marriage involves no danger for the man, but parturition does involve danger for the woman although far less than formerly. The danger is only slightly less than for the non-diabetic woman in similar physical condition. We have had some 1700 pregnancy cases of whom approximately 1200 have been under the supervision of Dr. Priscilla White. The infant survival after viability at first was 56 per cent but now is 87 per cent. Among these mothers, 2 have died of hepatitis within 3 months following delivery; 2 of coronary disease, one in the first trimester and the other after discharge from the hospital. There was one obstetrical death.

To reduce all hazards to the minimum, the pregnant diabetic should be under close observation and should enter a hospital for the last two weeks or more of pregnancy, certainly for the first child, and it is wiser under all circumstances. The condition of a diabetic woman during pregnancy may change suddenly and arrangements should be perfected early in its course so that she can be hospitalized at a moment's notice. With close observation neither she nor the doctor need have many worries. As late as 1885, Bouchardat, that noted French physician and the leading diabetes specialist of all time, said he could not remember having seen a pregnant diabetic woman. Today diabetics become pregnant as readily as non-diabetics.

When diabetes is controlled, diabetic complications of the disease in mother and infant are absent or rare, but the reverse holds for the uncontrolled diabetic. The babies of diabetics tend to be big. They are long and heavy. They are likely to be overweight, especially if the disease in the mother has been uncontrolled, and they are often waterlogged. Since they look unusually plump and so healthy, their strength is overestimated. Frequently in the past a mother has lost her child simply from the mechanical difficulty of its birth.

Complications can develop in the eyes, kidneys, arteries and nerves of the mother, particularly after the disease has lasted ten years or more. These conditions are quite apart from the danger of diabetic coma or insulin reactions which is ever present. Ability to beget healthy children, on the part of the father as well as the mother, also varies with the duration of the disease and its control. Consequently, diabetics should always plan for a family as soon as possible after marriage.

Cesarean section is frequently the type of delivery selected, not so much because of the size of the baby, but in order to anticipate toxemia which formerly was such an important factor in infant mortality. In general, this is done three to five weeks before term, because during these last few weeks toxemia may cause the death of the child. Today toxemia is far less inevitable, because often it can be prevented or controlled by medical means. The safety of the child is rapidly advancing with the application of new measures. A fetal survival of 56 per cent prior to 1936 has risen in 1958, in Dr. White's recent series, to 87 per cent.

The diet of a diabetic mother should contain about 200 grams of carbohydrate, because the foetus needs nearly 50 grams. The quantity of protein should be somewhat increased and fat should be regulated according to the weight of the patient. The total calories should not lead to undue gains in weight, because large babies should be avoided. This latter possibility is now more easily accomplished by the use of a low salt diet and appropriate medication. A minimum of 1 pint and often 1 quart of milk should form a part of the mother's diet. The use of female sex hormones in our experience has favored normal course and outcome.

During the pregnancy insulin may be doubled or trebled, but there is no increased severity of the disease afterwards. In none of the cases did disease of the eyes develop during the pregnancy, and progression of an existing retinitis when under careful management was rare. Disease of the kidneys was observed first in the pregnancy in only 2 cases, and an existing nephritis progressed in but 4 cases, and there was no progression shown during the pregnancy in 63 cases.

The hours immediately following delivery are critical

both for mother and child. Access to a laboratory in which tests for non-protein nitrogen, blood sugar, carbon dioxide combining power, and the blood chlorides can be performed either by day or by night, removes nearly all risks. Sudden alterations in the insulin requirements of the mother often follow delivery. The infant, too, must be watched, because generally it is a premature infant. It should be kept in an incubator and with minimal oxygen for the first few days. Usually it is a so-called wet baby and requires special attention to remove water from the air passages and to promote respiration. Food and water are usually contraindicated for a day or more for this reason. None of our babies has required glucose to offset a low blood sugar. The question of nursing the baby depends upon the ability of the mother to control her diabetes and maintain her strength and proper weight, but seldom is nursing desirable.

The importance of intimate cooperation between the physician and the obstetrician led to the inclusion of a delivery room in the George F. Baker Clinic of the New England Deaconess Hospital, but we have given it up, because we have found it safer to care for our patients at the time of delivery in the Boston Lying-In Hospital. The treatment of a pregnant diabetic begins at the earliest recognition of the pregnancy and lasts until a month after delivery. For success, visits at first to the physician and obstetrician should be every week. The most critical period for the infant is during the last five weeks of the pregnancy. Delivery has been by Cesarean section in 50 per cent of Dr. White's series.

It may seem to some that I am too frank in recording my ideas about the marriage of diabetics, but I believe such statements should be made. Particularly do I think this desirable when I see a non-diabetic boy or girl about to marry a diabetic whose disease has been uncontrolled for ten or fifteen years, because I know it is almost certain the latter will have serious complications in the eyes, kidneys or arteries of the heart, brain or legs within a decade resulting in prolonged periods of incapacity. These statements do not apply to the controlled diabetic. At times girls and boys marry although dangerous impairments exist, but this should be done only with the complete understanding of their presence and the willingness to accept the responsibilities and consequences.

If a diabetic marries a non-diabetic of a non-diabetic family, their children should escape unscathed, but of course all these children would be hereditary carriers and capable of transmitting the disease. However, unless they married persons who were also hereditary carriers, their own children would not develop diabetes.

A considerable number of our diabetics have married and later died. As yet the one left behind, or the family of the survivor, in no instance has blamed us for allowing the marriage to have taken place and we have been told that depsite the sadness a death caused (this held even before the discovery of insulin) all concerned were thankful that the marriage had occurred.

What is the effect of diabetes upon a race? (See p. 226.)

In any crusade against diabetes no consideration appears to be given to possible advances in the treatment or prevention of the disease. Even fifty years ago it was clear that progress in diabetes was imminent, because shortly before that time von Mering and Minkowski's discovery of diabetes following removal of the pancreas had been made and Opie's and Ssobolew's observation upon the relation of the islands of Langerhans to the disease had just been published. And what of today with the almost complete abolition of diabetic coma, the diminishing death rate in the young, the relative safety in operations, all of which have followed the discovery of insulin? Yet all of these past achievements seem insignificant when one realizes the better scientific weapons, the better fields for action in our laboratories and the greatly increased number of really skilled research workers, all now available for a successful attack on the disease. There was never a greater opportunity for the discovery of new methods of treatment of diabetes than today and he is certainly pessimistic who would forbid the marriage of diabetics upon the ground that advance in the therapy of diabetes had reached an impasse.

The danger of a pregnancy to a diabetic mother today is almost non-existent, because the patient is under constant control. Insulin washed clean the slate of the old rules for pregnant diabetics. Cesarean section is permissible with practically the same freedom from worry as in a non-diabetic, provided it is performed by skilled obstetricians working in association with doctors trained in the treatment of the disease.

A Cesarean section is justifiable because it is unlikely that diabetic mothers will have many children and it is therefore important to do everything to save each one.

Sterilization is a last resort and in our experience does more harm than good.

23

WEIGHT PECULIARITIES

NINE out of ten diabetics whose disease began after thirty years of age were overweight at some period of their lives. See Table 15, p. 215. If you are the relative of a diabetic and want to dodge diabetes, don't be fat! It is a great deal easier and more important to avoid overweight when young because thereby you may escape a lifetime of diabetes as well as degeneration of the blood vessels. As soon as sugar begins to be lost in the urine, the weight usually falls (even though the quantity of food be excessive) because the body is unable to utilize it. It is not uncommon for a patient to get fat a year or two before the diabetes is discovered and then to lose 50 pounds before treatment begins. Occasionally a patient will lose as much as 100 pounds during the course of years. A diabetic patient, whose urine is free from sugar, in reality is in safer condition if he is 10 to 25 per cent below weight, because then he knows he is not overeating. In this respect it is better to emulate the Navajo Indian and cartoonists' Uncle Sam than John Bull. Is the low percentage of diabetes in Great Britain today due to the reduction of the average body weight of the inhabitants? By losing weight a patient often regains the power to tolerate carbohydrate. As a guide to the proper weight for a diabetic the average weights of individuals for given heights and ages are given in Tables 17 to 21. Tables 22 and 23 take into account the bodily frame of the individual and in some respects are more reliable.

Gain in weight in the course of diabetes is usually encouraging, but the weight gained should be moderate and not quite sufficient to bring the weight of the patient up to normal standard. Even with insulin one sees the harmful effect of a marked gain in weight, because it is then more difficult to keep the urine sugar-free. It is a good rule to keep the weight a little below normal.

Changes in Weight During Treatment

Diabetic patients are often surprised at the sudden change in weight when they undergo a short course of treatment. It may go up or down 5 to 10 pounds in as many days. The reason for these queer changes is the

TABLE 17.—HEIGHTS AND WEIGHTS OF CHILDREN BETWEEN ONE AND FOUR YEARS OF AGE (WITHOUT CLOTHES).*

5602 Boys			4821 Girls	
Height, inches	*Weight, pounds*	*Age, months*	*Height, inches*	*Weight, pounds*
26.5	18.0	6	25.9	16.8
29.4	21.9	12	28.9	20.8
31.8	24.6	18	31.1	23.4
33.8	27.1	24	33.4	26.4
35.4	29.5	30	34.9	28.3
37.1	32.3	36	36.8	30.5
38.6	33.8	42	38.0	32.5
39.5	35.9	48	39.0	33.8

* Crum, F. S.: Quarterly Publications of the American Statistical Association, Boston, September, 1916, N. S., No. 115, *15*, 332.

retention or discharge of water from the tissues. Weigh yourself and drink two glasses of water and see how much you gain, or weigh yourself before and after a meal. The following experiment conducted by me many years ago illustrates this well: A healthy student was given a diet sufficient to maintain his body weight so far as nutritive value was concerned, but from his food salt was entirely removed.[1] As a result, in the course of

[1]The diet was strictly salt-free and consisted of rock candy, and whites of eggs, boiled, and olive oil, the latter two being washed free of salt.

thirteen days the weight fell 12 pounds. Upon the resumption of his former diet with salt as desired, 9 pounds of those lost were regained in three days. Diabetic patients often gain weight from exactly the same cause—namely, the ingestion of too much salt. Such gain in weight, however, should be looked upon at its face value, in other words simply as a retention of fluid in the body.

TABLE 18.—HEIGHTS AND WEIGHTS OF BOYS BETWEEN FIVE TO FOURTEEN YEARS (WITHOUT CLOTHES).[1]

AGE	3-3	3-4	3-5	3-6	3-7	3-8	3-9	3-10	3-11	4	4-1	4-2	4-3	4-4	4-5	4-6	4-7	4-8	4-9	4-10	4-11	5	5-1	5-2	5-3	5-4	5-5	5-6	5-7	5-8
5		35	38	39	41	42	46																							
6		38	39	41	42	44	46	48																						
7				42	43	46	48	49	54																					
8						45	48	50	53	54	57	59																		
9								50	53	55	58	60	62	62	65															
10									53	55	58	60	62	65	68	69	71													
11													61	61	65	68	71	77	77	78										
12														63	67	70	75	76	79	84	84	85								
13															67	71	75	78	80	85	86	91	98	99	100					
14															67	71	76	79	82	86	90	94	97	103	107	114	122			
15																		79	82	87	91	95	99	106	112	118	119	121	128	133

TABLE 19.—HEIGHTS AND WEIGHTS OF GIRLS BETWEEN FIVE TO FOURTEEN YEARS (WITHOUT CLOTHES).[1]

AGE	3-3	3-4	3-5	3-6	3-7	3-8	3-9	3-10	3-11	4	4-1	4-2	4-3	4-4	4-5	4-6	4-7	4-8	4-9	4-10	4-11	5	5-1	5-2	5-3	5-4	5-5
5		34	37	38	41	41	45																				
6			35	37	39	41	43	45	48																		
7					39	42	44	45	47	50																	
8						42	45	47	49	51	53	56															
9								49	51	53	56	59	63														
10										54	57	58	62	64	69												
11												60	62	63	68	70	75										
12													63	66	69	71	75	78	83	88	94						
13														65	68	73	76	80	86	89	94	99	104				
14																		78	83	88	93	96	100	104	107	112	114
15																				89	97	100	102	106	109	118	118

[1]Wood, T.D.: The ninth yearbook of the National Society for the Study of Education, Part I, Health and Education, Chicago, 1910, p. 34.

TABLE 20.—HEIGHTS AND WEIGHTS OF 221,819 MEN OF FIFTEEN OR MORE YEARS OF AGE (WITH CLOTHES).[1]

Graded average weight in pounds with clothes.

Feet and inches with shoes.

Age	5-0	5-1	5-2	5-3	5-4	5-5	5-6	5-7	5-8	5-9	5-10	5-11	6-0	6-1	6-2	6-3	6-4	6-5
15	107	109	112	115	118	122	126	130	134	138	142	147	152	157	162	167	172	177
16	109	111	114	117	120	124	128	132	136	140	144	149	154	159	164	169	174	179
17	111	113	116	119	122	126	130	134	138	142	146	151	156	161	166	171	176	181
18	113	115	118	121	124	128	132	136	140	144	148	153	158	163	168	173	178	183
19	115	117	120	123	126	130	134	138	142	146	150	155	160	165	170	175	180	185
20	117	119	122	125	128	132	136	140	144	148	152	156	161	166	171	176	181	186
21	118	120	123	126	130	134	138	141	145	149	153	157	162	167	172	177	182	187
22	119	121	124	127	131	135	139	142	146	150	154	158	163	168	173	178	183	188
23	120	122	125	128	132	136	140	143	147	151	155	159	164	169	175	180	185	190
24	121	123	126	129	133	137	141	144	148	152	156	160	165	171	177	182	187	192
25	122	124	126	129	133	137	141	145	149	153	157	162	167	173	179	184	189	194
26	123	125	127	130	134	138	142	146	150	154	158	163	168	174	180	186	191	196
27	124	126	128	131	134	138	142	146	150	154	158	163	169	175	181	187	192	197
28	125	127	129	132	135	139	143	147	151	155	159	164	170	176	182	188	193	198
29	126	128	130	133	136	140	144	148	152	156	160	165	171	177	183	189	194	199
30	126	128	130	133	136	140	144	148	152	156	161	166	172	178	184	190	196	201
31	127	129	131	134	137	141	145	149	153	157	162	167	173	179	185	191	197	202
32	127	129	131	134	137	141	145	149	154	158	163	168	174	180	186	192	198	203
33	127	129	131	134	137	141	145	149	154	159	164	169	175	181	187	193	199	204
34	128	130	132	135	138	142	146	150	155	160	165	170	176	182	188	194	200	206
35	128	130	132	135	138	142	146	150	155	160	165	170	176	182	189	195	201	207
36	129	131	133	136	139	143	147	151	156	161	166	171	177	183	190	196	202	208
37	129	131	133	136	140	144	148	152	157	162	167	172	178	184	191	197	203	209
38	130	132	134	137	140	144	148	152	157	162	167	173	179	185	192	198	104	210
39	130	132	134	137	140	144	148	152	157	162	167	173	179	185	192	199	205	211
40	131	133	135	138	141	145	149	153	158	163	168	174	180	186	193	200	206	212
41	131	133	135	138	141	145	149	153	158	163	168	174	180	186	193	200	207	213
42	132	134	136	139	142	146	150	154	159	164	169	175	181	187	194	201	208	214
43	132	134	136	139	142	146	150	154	159	164	169	175	181	187	194	201	208	214
44	133	135	137	140	143	147	151	155	160	165	170	176	182	188	195	202	209	215
45	133	135	137	140	143	147	151	155	160	165	170	176	182	188	195	202	209	215
46	134	136	138	141	144	148	152	156	161	166	171	177	183	189	196	203	210	216
47	134	136	138	141	144	148	152	156	161	166	171	177	183	190	197	204	211	217
48	134	136	138	141	144	148	152	156	161	166	171	177	183	190	197	204	211	217
49	134	136	138	141	144	148	152	156	161	166	171	177	183	190	197	204	211	217
50	134	136	138	141	144	148	152	156	161	166	171	177	183	190	197	204	211	217
51	135	137	139	142	145	149	153	157	162	167	172	178	184	191	198	205	212	218
52	135	137	139	142	145	149	153	157	162	167	172	178	184	191	198	205	212	218
53	135	137	139	142	145	149	153	157	162	167	172	178	184	191	198	205	212	218
54	135	137	139	142	145	149	153	158	163	168	173	178	184	191	198	205	212	219
55	135	137	139	142	145	149	153	158	163	168	173	178	184	191	198	205	212	219

[1] Association of Life Insurance Directors and Actuarial Society of America, New York, 1912, p. 38. Published by a committee. Allow 1 inch for shoes and 10 pounds for clothes.

TABLE 21.—HEIGHTS AND WEIGHTS OF 136,504 WOMEN OF FIFTEEN OR MORE YEARS OF AGE (WITH CLOTHES).[1]

| Age | Graded average weight in pounds with clothes. Feet and inches with shoes. | | | | | | | | | | | | | | | | |
	4–8	4–9	4–10	4–11	5–0	5–1	5–2	5–3	5–4	5–5	5–6	5–7	5–8	5–9	5–10	5–11	6–0
15	101	103	105	106	107	109	112	115	118	122	126	130	134	138	142	147	152
16	102	104	106	108	109	111	114	117	120	124	128	132	136	139	143	148	153
17	103	105	107	109	111	113	116	119	122	125	129	133	137	140	144	149	154
18	104	106	108	110	112	114	117	120	123	126	130	134	138	141	145	150	155
19	105	107	109	111	113	115	118	121	124	127	131	135	139	142	146	151	155
20	106	108	110	112	114	116	119	122	125	128	132	136	140	143	147	151	156
21	107	109	111	113	115	117	120	123	126	129	133	137	141	144	148	152	156
22	107	109	111	113	115	117	120	123	126	129	133	137	141	145	149	153	157
23	108	110	112	114	116	118	121	124	127	130	134	138	142	146	150	153	157
24	109	111	113	115	117	119	121	124	127	130	134	138	142	146	150	154	158
25	109	111	113	115	117	119	121	124	128	131	135	139	143	147	151	154	158
26	110	112	114	116	118	120	122	125	128	131	135	139	143	147	151	155	159
27	110	112	114	116	118	120	122	125	129	132	136	140	144	148	152	155	159
28	111	113	115	117	119	121	123	126	130	133	137	141	145	149	153	156	160
29	111	113	115	117	119	121	123	126	130	133	137	141	145	149	153	156	160
30	112	114	116	118	120	122	124	127	131	134	138	142	146	150	154	157	161
31	113	115	117	119	121	123	125	128	132	135	139	143	147	151	154	157	161
32	113	115	117	119	121	123	125	128	132	136	140	144	148	152	155	158	162
33	114	116	118	120	122	124	126	129	133	137	141	145	149	153	156	159	162
34	115	117	119	121	123	125	127	130	134	138	142	146	150	154	157	160	163
35	115	117	119	121	123	125	127	130	134	138	142	146	150	154	157	160	163
36	116	118	120	122	124	126	128	131	135	139	143	147	151	155	158	161	164
37	116	118	120	122	124	126	129	132	136	140	144	148	152	156	159	162	165
38	117	119	121	123	125	127	130	133	137	141	145	149	153	157	160	163	166
39	118	120	122	124	126	128	131	134	138	142	146	150	154	158	161	164	167
40	119	121	123	125	127	129	132	135	138	142	146	150	154	158	161	164	167
41	120	122	124	126	128	130	133	136	139	143	147	151	155	159	162	165	168
42	120	122	124	126	128	130	133	136	139	143	147	151	155	159	162	166	169
43	121	123	125	127	129	131	134	137	140	144	148	152	156	160	163	167	170
44	122	124	126	128	130	132	135	138	141	145	149	153	157	161	164	168	171
45	122	124	126	128	130	132	135	138	141	145	149	153	157	161	164	168	171
46	123	125	127	129	131	133	136	139	142	146	150	154	158	162	165	169	172
47	123	125	127	129	131	133	136	139	142	146	151	155	159	163	166	170	173
48	124	126	128	130	132	134	137	140	143	147	152	156	160	164	167	171	174
49	124	126	128	130	132	134	137	140	143	147	152	156	161	165	168	172	175
50	125	127	129	131	133	135	138	141	144	148	152	156	161	165	169	173	176
51	125	127	129	131	133	135	138	141	144	148	152	157	162	166	170	174	177
52	125	127	129	131	133	135	138	141	144	148	152	157	162	166	170	174	177
53	125	127	129	131	133	135	138	141	144	148	152	157	162	166	170	174	177
54	125	127	129	131	133	135	138	141	144	148	153	158	163	167	171	174	177
55	125	127	129	131	133	135	138	141	144	148	153	158	163	167	171	174	177

[1] Association Life Insurance Directors and Actuarial Society of America, New York, 1912, p. 67. Published by a committee. Allow 1½ inches for shoes and 6 pounds for clothes.

(239)

TABLE 22.—DESIRABLE WEIGHTS FOR MEN OF AGES 25 AND OVER
(Weight in Pounds According to Frame (as ordinarily dressed.)

Height (with shoes on)		Small Frame	Medium Frame	Large Frame
Feet	Inches			
5	2	116–125	124–133	131–142
5	3	119–128	127–136	133–144
5	4	122–132	130–140	137–149
5	5	126–136	134–144	141–153
5	6	129–139	137–147	145–157
5	7	133–143	141–151	149–162
5	8	136–147	145–156	153–166
5	9	140–151	149–160	157–170
5	10	144–155	153–164	161–175
5	11	148–159	157–168	165–180
6	0	152–164	161–173	169–185
6	1	157–169	166–178	174–190
6	2	163–175	171–184	179–196
6	3	168–180	176–189	184–202

TABLE 23.—DESIRABLE WEIGHTS FOR WOMEN OF AGES 25 AND OVER.
(Weight in Pounds According to Frame (as ordinarily dressed.)

Height (with shoes on)		Small Frame	Medium Frame	Large Frame
Feet	Inches			
4	11	104–111	110–118	117–127
5	0	105–113	112–120	119–129
5	1	107–115	114–122	121–131
5	2	110–118	117–125	124–135
5	3	113–121	120–128	127–135
5	4	116–125	124–132	131–142
5	5	119–128	127–135	133–145
5	6	123–132	130–140	138–150
5	7	126–136	134–144	142–154
5	8	129–139	137–147	145–158
5	9	133–143	141–151	149–162
5	10	136–147	145–155	152–166
5	11	139–150	148–158	155–169

These tables are based on numerous Medico-Actuarial studies of hundreds of thousands of insured men and women.

Printed by permission of the Metropolitan Life Insurance Company.

When water collects in excess in the body it is termed dropsy. Frequently this can be relieved and the patient lose weight by restricting the intake of salt, although not to the degree practiced in my experiment. On the other hand, preceding diabetic coma, there is a marked loss of weight. The body dries up and one of the chief aims in treatment is to correct this. Salt solution subcutaneously or intravenously is then almost always indicated in addition to water by mouth. It is not uncommon for a coma patient to gain 5 pounds overnight during treatment. One patient was given eleven quarts (22 pounds) of fluid in twelve hours and recovered. So, too, in diarrhea the desiccation of the tissues may be considerable.

A man or woman shudders at the thought of carrying about in his or her hands a bucketful of water—16 pounds—or, still more, a gallon of liquid in the form of dropsy, but how many ladies and gentlemen transport with composure several buckets of fat! They are not waterlogged, but fatlogged. Few of them are willing to face the elemental truth that no farmer has yet found a way to fatten hogs except with excess of food and little exercise. I fear I am a little hard-hearted toward my obese friends. A New England conscience compels the disclosure that my grandfather weighed 300 pounds, did not have diabetes, and death came from the old man's friend, pneumonia, upon his eightieth birthday. He was the exceptional man and to him I attribute my optimism which is so helpful in medicine.

Removal of the carbohydrate in an individual's diet, though it is replaced by an equivalent number of calories in the form of fat, causes a prompt fall in weight, and if the reverse procedure is adopted, the weight will rise. The loss or gain of weight which occurs under such conditions may amount to 2 pounds in a day for several days. It is explained by the varying quantities of water which are retained in the body according to whether carbohydrate or fat is stored.

Finally, there is a real reason for a loss of weight during the treatment of diabetes, aside from the loss of food in the form of sugar in the urine. It is due to the fact that at times the diet is deficient in calories. Under such circumstances the patient lives upon his own tissues. Calculations show that in this way there is an equivalent of about 1500 calories for every pound lost. To gain or lose 1 pound of actual tissue, therefore, there must be, approximately, an excess or deficit of 1500 calories. If a patient, therefore, is taking just the proper quantity of food for his daily needs and gains 1 pound, the discriminating doctor knows it simply means retention of water.

Sudden change in weight due to expulsion of sugar from the blood and retention of water may temporarily affect vision. Therefore, at the beginning of treatment, wait a few weeks until the eyes accommodate to this before being fitted for glasses.

If a loss of weight is not explainable diabetically, then one hunts for other reasons—exophthalmic goiter, tuberculosis, malignant disease.

If a diabetic wishes to lose weight, he can do so easily if the total calories in the diet are reduced. He simply eats less of everything, particularly of fat foods, because fat is a concentrated food, contains, gram for gram, double the calories of protein or carbohydrate and so will be missed the least. Such a diabetic diet is usually attainable by the omission of cream, bacon, oil, cheese, except for skimmed milk cheese, limitation of butter to a teaspoonful at a meal, and avoidance of fat meats and fish or obvious fat on the same, all the time being careful not to replace the decrease of fat by an increase of carbohydrate. The basic diet minus butter, Table 2, page 62 will serve as a guide.

If an individual lives on such a diet the weight will

fall, but it may not show the first few days and will not show if water is retained.

Don't take drugs to help lose weight. Depend upon your own backbone and self-control. It is a life-saving procedure to overcome obesity and it pays. It is encouraging that the lowered life expectancy which over-weight causes can be reversed if weight is lowered.

24

DOGS, DIABETICS AND THEIR FRIENDS

A DOG is a diabetic's thoughtful friend.

A dog never says to a diabetic "You are thin," never speaks about his diet, never tempts him to break it and to eat a little more, never refers to the delicacies he himself has eaten or the good bones he expects to eat, in fact never implies by any signs or action in public or in private that he knows his master has diabetes. A diabetic is never embarrassed by his dog. How often he wishes his friends were as considerate!

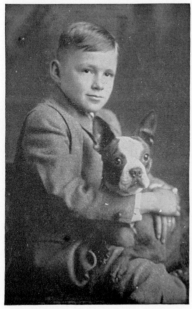

FIG. 32.—A diabetic child (Case 2007). George, a Cesarean at 8 months, was referred to me by Dr. John L. Morse, Professor of Children's Diseases, Harvard Medical School, in December, 1920, with 4.4% sugar at age of 4.8 years, was treated with temporary undernutrition and then with a relatively high carbohydrate diet and kept sugar-free until in 1923 insulin was begun, gradually increased to 80 units by 1933, but in 1953, 65 units. At first there was no diabetic heredity, but eventually two grandparents, a parent and aunt developed diabetes. Two children were born in 1943 and 1945. Diet has been followed with unusual care, disease controlled and no time lost from work on account of diabetes. Health excellent 1959. His wife is a nurse.

A dog is a diabetic's teacher. His dog shows the diabetic how to rest and sleep at odd moments, shows him how to exercise and play, recognizes the value of sunshine and sets him a good example by cleaning his paws every night. A dog is cheerful. The friends of a diabetic sometimes wish that he would take lessons from his dog.

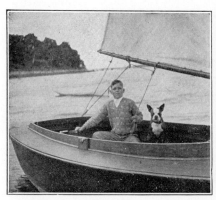 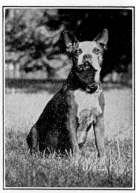

FIG. 33.   FIG. 34.

FIG. 33.—Case No. 2007. George with his crew, Bob, in 1926 has won many races. George is one of the diabetic children who is sailing unchartered seas to discover how older diabetics and other children can live. See Fig. 28, page 210.

FIG. 34.—Finally Bob died at the ripe old age, for a dog, of twelve years, equivalent to eighty-four years for a man. And what did George do? Why, of course—he married a nurse with a non-diabetic heredity and in 1959 they have two healthy children.

From experiments on a dog Minkowski found out that diabetes originated in the pancreas. From experiments on a dog Allen learned that undereating helped and overeating harmed diabetics. From experiments on a dog Banting and Best discovered insulin and Young produced experimental diabetes, which Best was able to prevent by keeping the blood sugar normal, thus for the first time foreshadowing the prevention of the disease in a human animal.

When I think of this little boy, George, and his dog, Bob, and their devotion to one another, I am reminded of the three million diabetics in the United States who may not be holding a dog in their arms, yet are alive today, enjoying better health and happiness, all because a few dogs through the instrumentality of multitudes of scientific workers have revolutionized the treatment of diabetes.

Would you want to be a member of a society if it had for its object the prevention of a dog saving the life of a child? Do you think this dog, Bob, would want to join such a society?

25

DIABETIC CHILDREN

Train up a child in the way he should go,
And when he is old he will not depart from it.

PROVERBS, 22:6.

THE diabetic child at the onset of his disease is usually taller and heavier, unless under modern treatment, than the average child and our tests showed him to be mentally precocious. When properly treated he grows and develops like a normal child. As a rule he has better teeth. The diabetic child I believe to be a superior being and I wish I could prove this to be true of the child of a diabetic.[1] Many disagree with my estimate, but I still adhere to it.[2] I think he is more gifted at birth and that his bringing up, if properly conducted, gives him self-confidence, a sense of responsibility and self-control and unusual knowledge. Environment, I agree, is an important factor.

Intelligence is inborn in the diabetic child. At the age of ten years he acquires a knowledge of diabetes far more readily than the average diabetic of fifty years. It is true he lacks judgment and has not learned to reason, largely because he has not had the opportunity to study in the school of experience. He knows his Benedict test and is well aware of its significance. He understands the reckoning of his diet and recognizes

[1] At a recent convocation for the award of Citations of Merit, I know that three of the six recipients had a diabetic parent, my Cases 8, 381 and 2903.

[2] The heights, weights and mortality of diabetic children should be re-investigated. Both weights and heights should be tabulated.

(247)

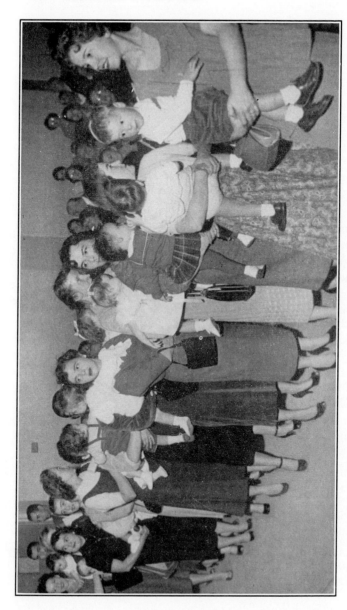

FIG. 35.—A Few of the 40 diabetic mothers and 75 babies waiting to be presented awards for their victory over diabetes at the fall public meeting of the Greater Boston Diabetes Society, Inc. (Diabetes Newsletter, 4, No. 4, February, 1959.)

errors in the same. He can administer his own insulin and occasionally prefers to do so. After a few experiences he detects the advent of an insulin shock almost intuitively. He appreciates what coma is, how it comes on, but is no more skillful in recognizing its stealthy approach than are nurses or most of us doctors.

Diabetic children are more sinned against than sinning and it is because of this that they do not get a fair show. They reflect their home training and their daily surroundings. They are underfed and overfed by a physician's fiat, often without rhyme or reason, because we do not take the time to study the individual cases and unearth their real needs. Some of us even have fads and may try to see on how little or, worse yet, on how much protein, carbohydrates or calories we can maintain their existence. Insulin and diet are so wonderful we are wont to dispense with our brains. The oral drugs, especially DBI, complicate the situation, but in the end I hope will solve it. We are generally more responsible than these little beings for their shortcomings, and if a doctor is frank, he will acknowledge it, hence this story.

Martin R., aged six years, came to the office, but was "just a naughty boy," according to a most experienced diabetic nurse, and to avoid a scene his parents took him home without his being met by me. When I heard of it, I upbraided all concerned and commented on the impropriety of a child dictating to his parents. Four hours later Martin returned smiling and it was suggested to me, supposedly versed in diabetic lore, that the fit of temper was simply due to an insulin reaction, because it had been easily cured by a few grams of carbohydrate. I was the bad boy and not the child. In such a case a psychiatrist is not needed, but a more wide-awake doctor.

Diabetic children mean to be honest. If they break a rule of diet, because they follow their instinct of self-preservation and sense of hunger, be careful what you say or do. If you say they steal food in their presence or before others, I protest and declare you are performing a criminal act before the bar of a child's soul if not before the bar of the law. Children eventually will tell whether they have done right or wrong, but don't force them to do so.

> "Do not rejoice when your enemy
> falls,
> and let not your heart be glad
> when he stumbles; . . ."
>
> PROVERBS 24:17

They will furnish the explanation of unexpected phenomena. Just as it is easier to be a total abstainer than a moderate drinker, so the old strict diet with starvation was easier to follow than the present liberal diets. Formerly diets were concrete; now they are intricate, and decision must be left to the judgment of the child to determine if he should eat the sugar you make him carry in his pocket to protect him from unconsciousness and convulsions because of an insulin reaction.

It is not so simple a matter to control the diet today as formerly. Then a slight error in diet showed instantly in the Benedict test, but now it is less apt to be a true indicator of what has been eaten, because of insulin and the larger meals, since moderate additions to the diet are often temporarily tolerated. The child sees you constantly testing his tolerance by addition to his carbohydrate and it is natural for him to test it too.

Never ask a diabetic child if he has broken his diet any more than you would ask your best friend if he had been dishonest. Never accuse any one of breaking his diet. Instead proceed in the plainest and most logical manner to seek the truth. Express wonder and surprise about what has happened. Together with the child search for the reason. Build up the evidence point by point without disclosing your intent or suggesting that you realize its convincing force until the child has no desire to do else than account for the enigma. But do not force him to put this in words. Recall Hawthorne's *Scarlet Letter* and the agony of Arthur Dimmesdale who wanted to confess, but was prevented from confessing. Never fear, the poor little child is punished enough by his own conscience and far more than if you had accused him. And when you are done with holding court, dismiss and forget the case.

A child lacks perspective so far as time is concerned. An hour is a day, a day is a week, a month a year and a year is eternity. Hence be cautious and use great discretion in discussions before children. If questions about the future are asked, they must be promptly answered. Of course no one expects that diabetes will be treated ten years from now as it is today. There are hundreds working upon diabetic problems at present for each investigator a generation ago and the chances of notable discoveries and improvements in treatment are infinitely better. I firmly believe that something will be found which will make those lazy islands of Langerhans secrete more and better insulin. In the meantime every diabetic who prolongs his life for one day is encouraging another to live bravely too.

Transgression of the diet is frequently the fault of the doctor and for one of two causes. Either the doctor (and of course here I am referring to myself) has not explained clearly enough to Johnnie the reason for recommending those strange and funny meals, which his mother never used to give him, or a regimen of diet, exercise and insulin has been planned which is incompatible with elementary principles of health.

The most important education for a diabetic child anyway is his diabetic education, because upon that his life depends. No matter how devoted the parents, no matter whether wealth allows a nurse, nothing will take the place of a child acquiring for himself the fundamentals of his disease and how to combat it success-fully. To do this, encourage association with other diabetic children so that their successes or failures will serve as examples.

Every diabetic child has his three mischievous ponies to drive and their names are Diet, Exercise and Insulin, just as are the diabetic horses of the adult diabetic. It is no joke for a child to manage one wilful pony, but a real struggle, and to harmonize the capriciousness of three such ponies is a tremendous triumph. To add an oral drug complicates the problem still more. The child must continually adjust the diabetic load between Diet, Exercise and Insulin, and he should not be discouraged despite frequent failures, because it can be done. Experience, the nurse, the doctor, and the parents and grandparents and brothers and sisters will finally bring success. I know whereof I speak because whereas in 1941 there were 24 of our children who had gone beyond twenty years of diabetes, now in 1958, of our 4219 children with onset under 15 years of age seen between 1897 and 1957, there are approximately 80 per cent, 3351, known to be alive. Of these, 8 have lived over 40 years; 75 over 35; 215 over 30; 689 over 25; 1241 over 20 years.

The lives of diabetic children should resemble as nearly as possible the lives of other children. Very likely it is better to graduate from the high school at eighteen or nineteen than at seventeen years. This will allow more time for exercise, broad reading and ma-turity.

The general health of diabetic children should be kept at its highest pitch. Sources of infection should be promptly removed. It is almost more important to remove an appendix, if there is a hint of trouble with it, than tonsils and teeth, because the symptoms of an appendicitis often resemble diabetic coma and both conditions may be coexistent. Children should be vaccinated against smallpox like any child and similarly protected against diphtheria and pneumonia. They can be inoculated against tetanus (lock-jaw) after the same preliminary testing which is employed for any child and have booster shots yearly, and also for polio.

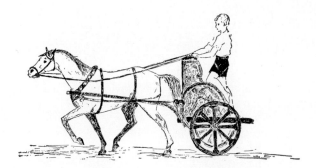

Fig. 36.—Diet is a steady steed.

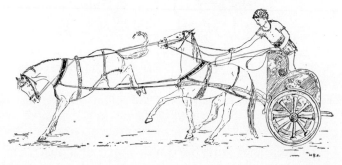

Fig. 37.—The performance of Diet and Exercise is not consistent.

Tuberculosis was once more common in diabetic children than in non-diabetic children but now has almost disappeared. This decline in tuberculosis opens up a nursing career for them, when they have proved their capacity to control their diabetes.

The diet of diabetic children is essentially the same as that of diabetic adults but greater in protein and calories for growth and activity. The food must be eaten slowly and the child must be in a rested state before meals. It is a mistake to pamper the appetites of children. Healthy children like plain foods and the same foods day after day. They love routine and habit. Mary's grandfather mischievously dropped a blueberry in the middle of the saucer of oatmeal Mary was contentedly eating and it spoiled her breakfast. It is a good plan for diabetic children or adults to make their breakfast a routine and take the carbohydrate later in the day. In this way no calculations are necessary for at least part of the meals.

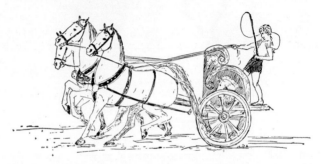

Fig. 38.—Diet and Exercise work together happily when harnessed with Insulin.

To keep pace with the development of diabetic children is not an easy undertaking. Not only must one be keen to discern gains in tolerance for carbohydrate, but one must provide for the all-around development of body, mind and soul. At puberty, especially, these children are unstable and require extra quantities of food. To deprive them then of an adequate diet leads either to their taking it for themselves or what is almost worse, namely, retarded development. One must keep abreast of their mental growth as well and direct them along channels where they can choose a suitable life's career. Between 12 and 20 years of age children eat more than at any other period of life and their insulin needs are the highest. Three months should never go by without having them report to a doctor in person or by letter or telephone. In fact, this is a good rule for all diabetics to follow. It is up to the doctor to make evident to patients that this is worth while—no light task for him.

Regular exercise is just as important as diet and insulin in the routine treatment of diabetic children.

Adolescent girls can be brought in line if they are in contact with a young mother and her baby or a young pregnant woman. The possibility of participation in athletics will help a boy to control his diabetes. These children are such delightful little indoor companions for their parents or caretakers that outdoor exercise is often overlooked. But remember that when the Exercise pony pulls hard, Diet and Insulin have less to do.

The diets of diabetic children, like those of ordinary children, should be more liberal than those of adults. During the year 1958 the camp diets of boys and girls were those shown in Table 24. In general I personally think their diets range too high rather than too low, but each individual case is a problem. What the future will disclose one can't predict, but all will study the diets of the Quarter Century Victory Medal cases.

We must follow up far more minutely our children and especially those at Camps where the treatment is less individualized. I am sure we should do more in detailed care of diabetic children than heretofore. They need a wandering diabetic nurse like a Miss Winterbottom, who 25 years ago helped in their homes.

Dr. Steinke who was in charge of the Elliott P. Joslin Camp in Charlton, Massachusetts during the 1958 season gives me the following table. Table 24, p. 256.

Coma is the chief danger which overhangs the diabetic child. Insulin reactions claim increasing attention, but diabetic coma ever will be the one condition which the child should thoroughly understand and be in a position to avoid. Prior to insulin practically all diabetic children died of coma. Today not one of them should die of coma. It is proof of neglect of diagnosis or of good treatment. After the duration of twenty years of diabetes, only 13 per cent of the children without a history of coma had trouble with their eyes, heart, kidneys and blood vessels, whereas of those incapacitated by these complications, 75 per cent had had coma repeatedly.

TABLE 24.—AVERAGE CAMP DIETS, 1958

Age Group Years	Carbohydrate Grams	Protein Grams	Fat Grams	Calories
5–7	150	80	65	1500
8–10	180	90	80	1800
11–12	200	100	90	2000
13–14	220	110	100	2200
15 and over	220	120	120	2400

The above diets include 4 lunches between meals as follows— varying with exercise.

1 snack at 10 a.m.	10 grams carbohydrate
1 snack at 2:30 p.m.	15 grams carbohydrate
1 snack at 3:30 p.m.	10 grams carbohydrate
1 snack at bedtime	10 grams carbohydrate

At the end of one week the patients were weighed and the diets adjusted accordingly.

Every child needs a "Buddy." His mother is his true friend when he is at home, but it is his Buddy who will look out for him at school, at college, and in play, and when so protected there is no form of athletics which he cannot pursue. Later, if he has a wise, devoted and loving wife, there is almost no limit to his future career.

Summer camps for diabetic children are splendid.[1] In 1940 we had 205 diabetic children distributed in five camps, and in 1958 in two camps we had 237 boys and 198 girls. The children have done wonderfully well, but the vacations have not been limited to the children, because their parents have profited by being relieved of their responsibility, often for the first time in years. Diabetic camps should be encouraged. Children are far more easily and naturally treated in them than in hospitals and at less expense. We are greatly indebted to The Association of Universalist Women which has made possible our camp for girls at the Clara Barton Birthplace in North Oxford, Massachusetts, where in 1821 Clara Barton, the founder of the Red Cross in the United States, was born. In 1947, our wish came true and, thanks to Dr. and Mrs. George G. Averill, we have the Elliott P. Joslin Camp for diabetic boys in Charlton, Massachusetts, three miles from the Clara Barton Camp. The children voluntarily contribute nearly one-half of the costs. Any large diabetic clinic for children should have access to such a camp. In the 1959 season there are 31 camps in operation in the United States and 6 in Canada, and the number all over the world is increasing.

All have recognized the advantages of diabetic camps. More of them are required but, with the lengthening of the lives of diabetic children, observations must be continued until the critical period of adolescence has been passed. I feel that the need today can be met by the establishment of Hospital Teaching Clinics, to which ambulatory diabetics can return often for a few days of orientation and rehabilitation of their physical condition before irremediable complications have been acquired. To meet this need hospitalization must be at far less than conventional hospital rates.

[1] For a list of Summer Camps for diabetic children, write American Diabetes Association, 1 East 45th Street, New York 17, New York.

17

Such a Hospital Teaching Clinic we have created under the auspices of Diabetes Foundation, Inc. and the success attending it has exceeded our greatest hopes.

The diabetic child should be taught hygiene and while he learns this for himself he should grasp its meaning so thoroughly that he will spread sound ideas among the rest of his family, and thereby make himself helpful in the home. If a child holds to his diet and insulin to control his diabetes, should not his relatives avoid being fat at forty or above and thus seek to escape it? The time may come when we may utilize these children more in medicine. Every diabetic unavoidably becomes a center of medical influence in his family. Every other one of my twenty-year duration diabetic children already has reported having a diabetic relative. One cannot begin too early teaching the child that a diabetic should choose a non-diabetic from a non-diabetic family for a partner in life.

Children love to assume responsibility. Trust them and they will carry out their duties well. Jane and Jeane lived 1500 miles apart, but their poor mothers were worn out. When Jane and Jeane were told this, their whole attitude changed and I had no more worry about those girls or about their mothers because I knew their children would compel them to take recreation and rests. Give any child, diabetic or otherwise, an opportunity to manage something or somebody and the chances are he or she will come out all right. They need to be given responsibility.

The morale of the diabetic child quite as much as that of the adult must be preserved. That is why I am so glad to learn of the success of those whose diabetes began in childhood and to report these to children whose diabetes is just commencing. Happily it is not difficult to maintain their spirits, because these children excel in school and in many sports. Occasions should be arranged in which they can show off and distinguish themselves.

Once upon a time diabetic children were pampered, but now their health so closely nears that of ordinary children that they must protect their own reputations. Just as no doctor is warranted in giving approval to a diabetic to drive an automobile if such a one carelessly has coma and insulin reactions, so, too, children must know that doctors take seriously their requests for recommendations for insurance and to college and business positions and can grant them only if they control their disease.

Each child who enters college or takes a job assumes a heavy responsibility and becomes accountable for his own conduct. Unless he does well, he will injure the prospects of admission to college or to similar jobs for hundreds of future young diabetics. To protect youthful diabetics, we have made the rule to recommend to college and institutions of higher learning diabetic boys and girls only on the condition that they will be physically examined monthly and their diabetic course checked by college medical authorities or those physicians selected by them. With this rule in force, we believe that distressing failures at college examinations can be avoided. Without such personal health surveys, diabetic boys and girls undoubtedly innocently have suffered in the past.

Sixty years ago when I began treating diabetic children I counted the days they lived. It is hard to believe, but it is true, that now the duration of the diabetes of some of these children has exceeded 40 years and it is evident soon will pass 50 years. Rigid control of the diabetes with rest to the islands of Langerhans by over insulination as described by Brush and many others often gives surprising results. Remissions may occur. Treasure them. Prolong them with close care and insulin. Who knows? One may have a reversible case.

26

TUBERCULOSIS

TUBERCULOSIS at one time caused the death of one-half of all those with diabetes. It is probably no exaggeration to say that this statement held for the hospital diabetic population in some crowded European cities even up to the discovery of insulin. Tuberculosis is still a deadly foe of the diabetic, particularly of those who are underprivileged. Fortunately, with earlier detection today and with new medical and surgical methods of treatment, it has dropped in 1957, as a cause of death in our own group to 0.2 per cent. Of the diabetics who had diabetic coma, it was found by Root and Bloor only a few years ago that more than one in five contracted tuberculosis within the subsequent five years, and still higher figures have been noted by other writers.

Control of the diabetes day in and day out and a routine detection x-ray of the chest yearly are the two best safeguards against tuberculosis.

27

NEURITIS (NEUROPATHY)

WHEN the diabetes is controlled, neuritis, a distressing affection of the nerves, seldom occurs. Usually it is preceded by months or years of neglected diabetes. Our Quarter Century Victory Medal cases are notably free from it and this has been the experience of all the authors who have carefully studied this condition. Unfortunately, control of diabetes is so often neglected that neuritis is a most frequent, distressing and often serious complication. Particularly does it occur in neglected diabetes of younger people.

Neuritis is most commonly accompained by pain, but may be manifested by other disturbances of sensation such as diminished perception of pain, numbness and burning. If the motor fibers of the nerves are involved, weakness of the muscles, resulting in local or general paralysis of the part may occur. Less commonly the digestive and urinary tracts may be involved. The duration of the symptoms may be quite temporary, disappearing soon after the blood sugar returns to a normal level; or they may be far more permanent, lasting for months, although eventually in large part they disappear. Complete recovery may take place in the most severe forms and we have several patients who are kind enough to return and attest their freedom from pain, although at one time almost one-hundred per cent crippled.

The most outstanding symptom of neuritis is pain which is characteristically worse at night. The extremities are most often affected. Pain may be superficial, deep, aching, grinding, darting or cutting. Paresthesiæ, such as burning, tingling, numbness, feeling as if walking on wool, "pins-and-needles" sensations, are frequent.

Occasionally just the opposite occurs and the skin is too sensitive—hyperesthesia. The weight of bed covers may be unbearable. Signs of neuritis are recognized by diminished or absent knee reflexes, by muscle tenderness, increased skin sensitivity to pin prick or the vibrations of the tuning fork, or the reverse, and by muscular weakness or even paralysis, and less commonly by rapid heart beating and lowered blood pressure with resulting dizziness or fainting on standing. If a muscle of the eye is affected, double vision results and may persist for six or more weeks.

The underlying cause of these complications in the nerves (neuritis), in the eyes (retinitis) and in the kidneys (nephritis) in diabetes may have a common origin. My colleague, Dr. Howard F. Root, groups the three under the term *triopathy*. Meticulous diabetic control we firmly believe will prevent, defer or ameliorate these complications. This combination is especially manifested in the uncontrolled diabetic of fifteen or more years' duration in whom the disease began under the age of forty years. Such cases were more rarely seen a generation ago, because patients lived so short a time. Even in older patients with relatively milder diabetes, numbness and tingling, particularly in the extremities, night pains, muscular weakness and impaired sensation may be encountered. As a result of the lessened sensitivity of the skin and inability to perceive pain, injuries to the skin leading to ulceration and sores are invited, particularly in the lower extremities. Such, if neglected, may lead to gangrene and to disintegration of the bones of the ankles and toes (Charcot joints). A most distressing complication in the digestive tract is nocturnal diarrhea and in the genito-urinary tract decreased potency and paralysis of the bladder. It is no wonder, therefore, that those of us who see these rarer complications are insistent that for their prevention diabetics should control their diabetes not only at the very start but through all the years.

28

COMPLICATIONS IN THE EYES

DIABETICS with perfect eyes after twenty-five years of diabetes are the exception. Those with sound eyes in our experience, are the individuals who have been under excellent control for the first few years of the disease and under good control always. It is seldom that a serious affection of the eyes is found or develops in the early days after the onset of diabetes, although occasionally the diabetes, long present, is first recognized by the eye specialist.

Troubles with the eyes are either temporary, relievable with control of the disease, or progressive and permanent. Temporary disturbances of refraction, resulting in impairment of vision, often appear in the first few days of treatment when the high percentage of sugar in the blood drops to normal. Eye specialists know this and patients should not seek to correct this temporary blurring of vision, because of itself it will largely disappear in a month and then there is either no need of glasses or a permanent adjustment can be made.

A distressing lesion is retinitis proliferans in which connective scar tissue extends out from the optic disc, the posterior portion of the retina, into the vitreous fluid which fills the globe of the eye. This is due to degenerative changes in the retina, manifested by exudates and hemorrhages. It is often associated with a peculiar disease of the kidney, described by Kimmelstiel and Wilson, and with neuritis and named diabetic triopathy by my colleague, Dr. Root. Bad as retinitis proliferans is, it is a hopeful complication, because it does not occur in those who control their diabetes. It is not like the changes resulting in the blood vessels from arteriosclerosis and high blood pressure.

Dr. Root has collected 847 instances of triopathy and undoubtedly there are many more. These have occurred especially in patients whose diabetes began in early life. There were 14 cases in the first two decades of life and 372 (43 per cent) in those who developed the condition before the age of 40 years, although the onset of diabetes occurs in only 33 per cent of our patients before that age.

Although the gravity of retinitis proliferans cannot be denied, it is true that in a considerable number of patients this complication remains stationary with respect to vision for lengthy periods. Long duration of diabetes and inadequate control of the condition were striking features in the great majority of cases. There was only one of these cases who had a history of careful treatment of diabetes, on the other hand, not one of our 85 Quarter Century Victory Medal cases showed it. No patient with excellent or good control of the diabetes showed advanced arterial calcification or retinitis even after periods of twenty-five years of diabetes.

Cataracts occur in diabetics as in non-diabetics, but whether they are more frequent is debatable. At any rate they are operable.

A few years ago, (1936), a serious disease attacked the eyes of premature babies, often leading to blindness. Indeed, even 33 per cent of our group of such babies, born several weeks before term, lost their eyesight or had it seriously impaired. It is a triumph of modern research that the cause of retrolental fibroplasia has been discovered and now several years may go by without an ophthalmologist seeing such a case. Research pays.

Just as there is common agreement that cigarettes are inadvisable in the presence of gastric or duodenal ulcer, neuritis or impaired circulation in the legs as a result of degeneration of the blood vessels, so too this holds in disease of the retina. At present it is safer for all diabetics to avoid cigarettes.

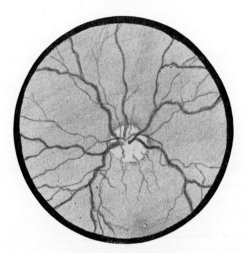

Fig. 39.—Normal eye.

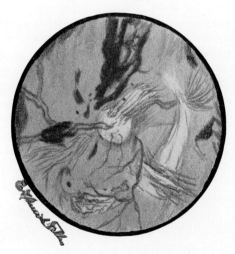

Fig. 40.—Retinitis Proliferans.

29

THE EMPLOYMENT OF DIABETICS—
INSURANCE FOR DIABETICS

THE Committee on Employment of Diabetics of the American Medical Association has issued the following statement: "Diabetics are capable of performing any type of work for which they are physically, mentally and educationally equipped. Those diabetics who are taking large doses of insulin should not, however, be assigned work in which hypoglycemic attacks might result in injury to themselves and others."

If a diabetic can secure employment which involves exercise, it is most advantageous, because exercise helps to utilize the diet and thus benefits the patient. If the employment does not involve exercise, then the diabetic must make up for it by taking exercise out of working hours. I remember well how those diabetics who progressed extraordinarily well in college while active in athletics, later when they graduated and took jobs, which did not involve exercise, such as postgraduate work in the law school or work in an office, found they did not do as well until they resumed exercise. Bouchardat was very insistent that his patients exercise until they sweated. He said they should earn their bread by the sweat of their brow, and they should use all the muscles of the body.

It is preferable for a diabetic to work independently and be his own master. Theoretically, a diabetic who is a farmer should do especially well, because he can regulate his exercise according to his work and need ask no questions of anyone.

Opportunities for employment of diabetics are many.

Particularly did this occur during World War II when they were given positions which did not involve combat activities. Today I understand that more than one thousand types of positions in the United States Civil Service are open to diabetics. I know of no argument stronger than what has occurred in our own group. Formerly it was seldom that more than one diabetic doctor, nurse, technician, secretary or camp counselor was employed by us, but in a recent summer seventeen diabetics held such paid positions. (I hope this statement will not result in a million diabetics applying to us for a job, because already we have quite a labor-diabetic pool of our own.)

Employers in general are kind to diabetics. It is very important that any diabetic seeking or holding an appointment should do his or her work not only as well but better than a non-diabetic in order to increase the opportunities for other diabetics to get a job. It is true a diabetic may need to give up certain pleasurable activities for the sake of securing and holding a good position, but if they can demonstrate their good health and their skill, then they will not need to fear.

Certain occupations are unsuitable for diabetics. Recently the American Diabetes Association has suggested standards for the employment of diabetics, and below I record abstracts from the same.

1. A diabetic seeking employment should be required to present a note from his physician or the personnel manager, stating that he is a controlled diabetic and is examined at regular intervals.

2. Diabetics are capable of performing any type of work for which they are physically, mentally and educationally equipped. Those diabetics who are taking large doses of insulin should not, however, be assigned work in which hypoglycemic attacks might result in injury to themselves and others.

3. An effort should be made to see that diabetics

work the same hours on a steady shift; or, if they must work on a rotating schedule, that they avoid the "graveyard" shift from midnight to 8 A.M. This is the only concession in terms of hours that a well-controlled diabetic should ask.

4. Diabetics should carry cards or tags identifying their condition at all times, particularly when on the job.

5. The plant physician can save time for the company and also help the employee by performing blood sugar and urine examinations, whenever the patient's usual laboratory facilities are available only during working hours, and the results reported to the family physician.

6. A complete physical examination of each diabetic should be made regularly, at least once a year.

7. A plant physician is within his rights if he re-assigns a diabetic employee to other work whenever the arising of new complications creates new risks for himself or for other employees.

8. The diabetic requiring insulin should be considered controlled if the fasting blood sugar is not below normal limits and not above 150 mg. per 100 cc. by the Folin-Wu method, and the blood sugar three hours after a meal is not higher than 250 mg. per 100 cc. by the Folin-Wu method, and if the patient is under regular medical supervision. Although more nearly normal blood sugar levels are desirable, hyperglycemia alone, if not extreme or habitual, need not be considered a disqualification for employment in those cases where the patient's personal physician and the industrial physician both feel that other limits should be observed.

Naturally, if diabetics have frequent reactions or develop diabetic coma, their chances for continuance in their occupation or for promotions are lessened. In a way this is fortunate, because it forces diabetics to study their diabetes thoroughly and to control it.

INSURANCE FOR DIABETICS

Until 1940 practically no known diabetic was granted insurance. At that time the Manufacturers Life Insurance Company in Toronto, Canada, undertook to insure diabetics. Gradually this company has increased the number insured and has broadened its policies and at lessened premiums. Its example has been followed generally, so that now approximately 75 per cent of all life insurance companies in the United States and Canada will accept diabetics on various terms.

The *chief* condition upon which insurance companies accept diabetics is proof that they are *under medical supervision*. Naturally all conditions which apply to non-diabetics apply to diabetics, but this one feature is apparently considered of more importance to the insurance company than detailed reports of tests for sugar in the urine and blood. Individually and collectively, the longer diabetics live without complications, the more likely are they to receive insurance on favorable terms.

30

AMERICAN DIABETES ASSOCIATION, INC.* AND INTERNATIONAL DIABETES FEDERATION

THE Association was founded and incorporated in 1940. Its objectives are to: 1. Disseminate among physicians information relative to the diagnosis and treatment of diabetes; 2. Educate the laity in the early recognition of diabetes, and in the importance of medical supervision; 3. Encourage and support clinical, experimental, sociological and statistical studies by means of grants; 4. Encourage adequate treatment of diabetes and the establishment of summer camps for diabetic children.

As of February 7, 1959, the American Diabetes Association had a total membership as follows: Active Members, 2421; Honorary Members, 10; Associate Members, 45; Corporate Members, 24; total 2500. There are members in every state of the union except Alaska and in forty-four foreign countries.

Allied with the American Diabetes Association are forty-two affiliate associations in the United States, supporting nationally and locally the objectives of the parent organization. Thirty-two of these affiliate associations have lay groups.

The Association publishes for the layman a bimonthly magazine, A.D.A. FORECAST; for the profession a bimonthly journal, DIABETES: The Journal of the American Diabetes Association. The Association keeps a list of diabetes camps.

*1 East 45th Street, New York City 17, N. Y.

The year-round detection program culminating in Diabetes Week accelerates the mass scale screening of individuals for diabetes. It also calls country-wide attention to diabetes and strengthens the continuing activities of local physicians in testing as many as possible in the community for diabetes.

International Diabetes Federation

The International Diabetes Federation was organized in Holland in 1952. Fifteen countries were represented. The Second Congress was held in Cambridge, England in 1955, and the Third Congress in Düsseldorf, West Germany, in 1958. At this Congress 42 countries and all continents were represented by doctors or lay delegates. The attendance reached nearly 1800 persons. The President of the Federation for 1959, is Professor J. P. Hoet, of Louvain, Belgium, and the Executive Secretary is Mrs. R. Frank, 152 Harley Street, London W. I., England.

31

SELECTED LABORATORY TESTS USEFUL IN DIABETIC TREATMENT

An early diagnosis in diabetes is as important as in tuberculosis and is far more easily made. The disease usually begins insidiously and its prompt detection depends upon the routine examination of the urine of everybody rather than upon the examination of the urine of patients who present symptoms of the disease. General practitioners should teach all their patients, as a matter of routine, to have their own urines and the urines of the members of their families examined each birthday. Diabetes is an hereditary disease and therefore each diabetic should protect his grandparents, his parents, brothers and sisters and children by making a yearly examination of the urine and a semi-annual examination, if the relative is over forty years of age. Every boy and girl who studies chemistry should be taught how to test the urine for sugar.

The Metropolitan Life Insurance Company was kind enough to analyze my cases. The study showed that the mortality for cases of diabetes discovered by examination for life insurance and thus presumably early cases was much lower than for those discovered otherwise.

The mere presence of sugar in the urine does not warrant a diagnosis of diabetes. To prove diabetes exists a test for the blood sugar should be made. If the blood sugar percentage reaches 0.13 (130 mg.) fasting or 0.17 (170 mg.) venous blood after food with the Folin-Wu test or 110 mg. and 150 mg. respectively with the "true" glucose method (Smogyi-Nelson method) with sugar in the urine, diabetes usually can be assumed to be present. Borderline values are often inconclusive and therefore the test should be repeated after a few weeks or months.

Although diabetic patients can test their own urines for sugar, it is safer for all diabetic patients to check their own tests occasionally with those made by their physician.

The Collection of Urine

To collect the twenty-four-hour quantity of urine, discard that voided at 7 A.M. and then save in a cool place all urine passed thereafter up to and including that obtained at 7 A.M. the next morning. As a preservative a teaspoonful of xylol can be placed in the bottle before the collection of the urine.

It has become increasingly important since the advent of insulin at times to examine separately the urine voided before or after meals and on retiring and rising. If sugar is found in the twenty-four-hour urine one can learn by a study of the morning, afternoon, evening and night specimens whether this occurs uniformly throughout the entire day or at a single period. If the latter is the case, an investigation will disclose whether (*a*) an excess of carbohydrate has been taken at the previous meal; (*b*) the amount of insulin has been inadequate, because of (1) insufficient quantity, (2) faulty administration due to repeated injections in a single area of the body or to the interval before the meal being too short or (*c*) lack of exercise. When sugar is found in all four specimens of urine the total diet including carbohydrate should be lowered, insulin raised and sometimes exercise increased. The question of increase or decrease in exercise, however, depends upon various factors such as the existence of an intercurrent infection, which of itself usually brings back sugar in the

18

urine. The bedridden patient without fever should always take bed gymnastics.

Two Specimen Tests

If a separate specimen of urine is voided, half an hour after the rising specimen, a true idea of the presence or absence of sugar in the fasting state is obtained. This is very desirable for those patients taking both regular and protamine zinc insulin before breakfast. The 7 A.M. specimen represents the specimen which has been collecting for hours during the night in the bladder; the 7:30 or 8:00 A.M. specimen represents urine recently secreted and is therefore a better index of the sugar in the blood. By this second specimen test one can decide whether the doses of protamine zinc insulin, NPH, Lente and Globin insulin are correct. Tests during the day gauge the dosage of crystalline or regular insulin. (See Fig. 15, p. 139.)

Examination of the Urine for Sugar

The urines of healthy individuals and of carefully treated diabetics do not show sugar by the routine Benedict test for sugar. Sugar can be demonstrated readily if it amounts to as little as 0.08 per cent, and it may rise to as high as 9 or 10 per cent when the diabetic diet is not followed. Most untreated cases show between 2 and 6 per cent of sugar. The total quantity of sugar in the urine in the twenty-four hours is easily estimated by multiplying the percentage of sugar which the urine contains by the total amount of urine voided. Thus, if the total quantity of urine is 3000 cc. (1 quart equals 946 cc. and for rough calculations can be considered equal to 1000 cc. or 1 liter) and the percentage of sugar is 4 per cent, the amount of sugar in the urine would be (3000 by 0.04) 120 grams, that is, approximately 4 ounces or ¼ pound. (See p. 202.) It is not very often that one finds more than 1 pound of sugar excreted in the urine during twenty-four hours. The food value of sugar lost, if only 120 grams, is considerable. Each gram of sugar is equivalent to 4 calories, and 120 grams would amount to 480 calories in a day. This is one-fourth of the total food value required by an individual with a quiet occupation who weighs 60 kilograms (132 pounds). A diabetic therefore can be a food spendthrift.

Patients and doctors should calculate far more often than they are accustomed to do the total quantity of sugar lost in the urine for comparison with the diet.

The Benedict Test for Sugar

Many tests for sugar in the urine are employed. The Benedict test[1] is the best. The solution has the advantage of not decomposing, even after months.

The test is carried out as follows: Four drops of the urine to be examined are placed in a test-tube and to this are added 2.5 cc. (an ordinary teaspoon holds about 5 cc.) of Benedict's solution. The tube is shaken to mix the urine and solution and then placed in water that is already boiling. After being in the boiling water for five minutes the tube is removed and examined for evidence of sugar. In the presence of sugar the entire body of the solution will be filled with a precipitate, which may be greenish, yellow or red in color, according to whether the amount of sugar is slight or considerable. If the solution remains clear, the urine being tested is sugar-free; if one can read print through the solution the percentage of sugar is so slight that it can be disregarded; if a heavy greenish precipitate forms, it usually means there is a trace of sugar; the appearance of a yellow sediment indicates the presence of a few tenths per cent of sugar in the urine, and a red sediment more than 2 per cent. The colors should be read after

[1]Benedict, S. R.: Jour. Am. Med. Assn., *57*, 1193, 1911.

shaking thoroughly. If the mixture of urine and solution is to be heated over a free flame, then 8 drops of urine and 5 cc. of Benedict solution should be employed.

Upon removal from the boiling water shake the test-tube. A discoloration which occasionally forms upon the surface is unimportant and with shaking disappears.

If doubt arises in the patient's mind about the reliability of his Benedict's solution, he can test it by performing the usual test for sugar but substituting 4 drops of orange juice for urine, a drop or two of a grape, or even as little as $\frac{1}{16}$ of a raisin. The test with orange juice changes the Benedict solution to a bright red color.

Convenient methods for testing the urine for sugar are sold under the names of Clinitest, Clinistix and Tes-Tape.

Quantitative Tests for Sugar in the Urine

It is one of the chief advantages of modern treatment that the need for these tests is greatly reduced. The simplification of the treatment of diabetes means everything to the practitioner and patient. At the beginning of treatment, however, it is desirable to follow the reduction of sugar excreted along with changes of the diet and the determination of the percentage of sugar. Later on the aim should be to keep the urine practically sugar-free.

In our laboratory we use the Sumner Test for Dextrose. The procedure is as follows: 5 mg. of Dinitrosalicylic acid salt solution and 0.1 mg. of urine mixed in a test tube; boil for 3 minutes; cool and read in a photoelectric colorimeter.

Methods for the Determination of the Urinary Acids. Qualitative Tests

Diacetic Acid (CH_3COCH_2COOH). The simplest method for the detection of acidosis by urinary exam-

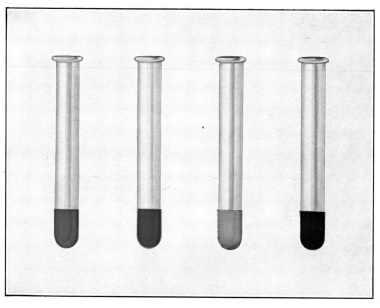

None.   Trace.   About 1%.   Over 2%.

THE BENEDICT TEST FOR SUGAR IN THE URINE

ination is Gerhardt's ferric chloride reaction for diacetic acid. The test may be performed as follows: To about 10 cc. of the fresh urine carefully add a few drops of an undiluted aqueous solution of ferric chloride, Liquor Ferri Chloridi, U.S.P. A precipitate of ferric phosphate first forms, but upon the addition of a few more drops is dissolved. The depth of the Burgundy red color obtained is an index to the quantity of diacetic acid present. Record the intensity of the reactions as follows: $+$, $++$, $+++$, or $++++$.

Confusion as to the significance of the test arises if the patient is taking sodium salicylate, aspirin, antipyrin, cyanates, or acetates. This is to a considerable extent avoided by vigorously boiling the urine after the addition of the ferric chloride, when the deep color markedly decreases or disappears if caused by diacetic acid, but remains the same if caused by the above drugs.

Acetone (CH_3COCH_3). The different tests for acetone are in reality tests for diacetic acid. Legal's test is as follows: A few crystals of sodium nitroprusside are dissolved in 5 cc. of urine, which is then rendered alkaline with sodium hydrate. Shake vigorously. Two drops of glacial acetic acid are then allowed to run down the side of the test-tube and a distinct purple color appears. A more convenient form is with a nitroprusside reagent, Acetest, which is for sale.

Tests for Blood Sugar

Blood sugar tests are essential in diagnosing diabetes and most valuable in treatment. Unfortunately, no method is available which is simple enough for patients to employ, but I suspect such will be discovered in the near future.

If tests for blood sugar are performed on a wholesale scale they are relatively cheap, but individual tests are expensive because it is almost as easy to do ten tests as one. An automatic method for blood sugar tests known as an "autoanalizer" is being introduced. With this apparatus a test requires but five minutes.

To reduce the cost of blood sugar tests one should find out what day and hour are the most convenient to the laboratory where they are to be performed. A "girl" doctor from Florida told me there were bargain blood sugar days in her city on which patients received a 60 per cent reduction. This is a sensible arrangement and I know is adopted in various laboratories. My suggestion is that a patient purchase a dozen blood sugar coupons wholesale from a hospital or laboratory yearly.

Blood sugar tests are extremely useful in treatment. Secure more of them! "Increase the output and lower the costs."

32

FOODS AND THEIR COMPOSITION

THERE is no one diet for all diabetics any more than there is one diet for all countries and races. If an individual avoids overweight or marked underweight the exact composition of the diet is relatively unimportant in health or in disease provided the diet is utilized and no sugar is lost in the urine. Without insulin in order to keep the urine sugar-free, most diabetics must restrict those foods which are rich in sugar and starch (carbohydrates) and make up for this restriction by eating more meat, fish, cheese and eggs (foods rich in protein) and fat. A patient can decide whether a given food is desirable by testing the urine one hour after eating it with or without his usual dose of insulin. F. M. Allen showed that a dog with much of his pancreas removed would develop diabetes most readily if overfed with carbohydrate, or with an excess of protein, and even with an excess of fat or alcohol.

The narrow confines of the diabetic diet in years past greatly stimulated the manufacture of so-called diabetic foods. These were often serviceable, but to be employed with discretion. The patient should never become dependent upon special diabetic foods, for they are often unobtainable, always make him conspicuous, and when he acquires a disgust for foods of this class it is all the harder to abide by the original diet. The patients under my care who have done best either never use special diabetic foods or use only a few varieties. Such foods should bear correct statements of the percentages of protein, fat, and carbohydrate which they contain; and under no circumstances should the label convey the impression that such foods may be eaten without restriction. See Table 26, pp. 287–296.

The high content of protein is one of the most serious drawbacks to diabetic foods. Formerly, when it was not realized that carbohydrate might be formed from protein, these special foods with low actual carbohydrate content were considered a great boon. Today we look at the matter differently.

We are indebted to Mrs. Elizabeth K. Caso, Nutritionist in the United States Public Health Service, for the preparation of the following dietary data.

METHOD OF CALCULATING
DIABETIC DIETS

A joint committee of the American Diabetes Association, American Dietetic Association, and Diabetes Section, United States Public Health Service, in 1950,[1,2] after 3 years of study, published a simplified method for calculating and planning diabetic diets. The data was approved by all three organizations. Since that time many hospitals and physicians throughout the country have used this information to guide and instruct diabetic patients concerning their diets. In brief the committee agreed upon the following figures for calculating diabetic diets. (Table 25 and pp. 280–286).

There are many ways by which patients may be taught the diet. Once in Vienna carbohydrate was reckoned according to the number of "semmels" a patient ate. In other centers one slice of bread has been the standard. With the varying composition of foods, both qualitative and quantitative, I have felt my pa-

[1] Revised Table of Food Values, Proc. Am. Diabetes A., *9*, 403, 1949.

[2] Caso: J. Am. Dietet. Assn., *26*, 575, 1950.

tients gained the most by weighing their food and calculating its content in carbohydrate, protein, fat and calories. This can be done readily by the use of Tables which I have combined on a pocket card. The American Diabetes Association and the American Dietetic Association have essentially the same basic diets but specify various exchanges. In a way I think this unfortunate, because actually the grams of carbohydrate, protein and fat are overlooked.

TABLE 25.—FOOD VALUES FOR CALCULATING DIABETIC DIETS

Group	Amount	Weight gm.	Car. gm.	Protein gm.	Fat gm.	Energy calories
Milk, whole (List 1)	½ pint	240	12	8	10	170
Vegetable (List 2A)	as desired	—	—	–	—	—
Vegetable (List 2B)	½ cup	100	7	2	—	36
Fruit (List 3)	varies	—	10	–	—	40
Meat Exchanges (List 4)	1 oz.	30	—	7	5	73
Bread Exchanges (List 5)	varies	—	15	2	—	68
Fat Exchanges (List 6)	1 tsp.	5	—	–	5	45

Foods of similar composition have been combined into "six food exchange lists." These lists are presented below:

Milk Exchanges List 1

One exchange contains: Carbohydrate 12 grams, protein 8 grams, fat, 10 grams: 170 calories

Amount to Use

Whole milk (plain or homogenized)..............	1 cup
*Skim milk....................................	1 cup
Evaporated milk............................	½ cup
Powdered whole milk........................	¼ cup
*Powdered skim milk (non-fat dried milk)........	¼ cup
Buttermilk (made from whole milk)............	1 cup
*Buttermilk (made from skim milk).............	1 cup

* Skim milk products contain less fat. When exchanged for whole milk add two fat exchanges to get the same food value.

Vegetable Exchanges List 2

Vegetable exchanges *A* contains: negligible amounts of carbohydrate, protein and fat. In raw form, size of serving unlimited; cooked, size serving ½ to 1 cup

Asparagus	*Escarole	Mustard greens	Sauerkraut
*Broccoli	Eggplant	Spinach	String beans, young
Brus. sprouts	GREENS	Turnip greens	Summer squash
Cabbage	Beet greens	Lettuce	*Tomatoes—1 per
Cauliflower	Chard	Mushrooms	serving
Celery	Collard	Okra	*Watercress
*Chicory	Dandelion	*Pepper	
Cucumbers	Kale	Radishes	

Vegetable exchanges *B* contains: carbohydrate 7 grams, protein 2 grams: 35 calories. One serving equals ½ cup.

Beets	Pumpkin
*Carrots	Rutabagas
Onions	*Squash, winter
Peas, green	Turnip

* Contains considerable amount of vitamin A.

Fruit Exchanges List 3

One exchange contains: carbohydrate 10 grams: 40 calories. Fruits may be fresh, dried, cooked, canned or frozen as long as no sugar is added.

	Amount to Use		*Amount to Use*
Apple (2" dia.)	1 small	Grapes	12
Applesauce	½ cup	Grape juice	¼ cup
Apricots, fresh	2 medium	Honeydew melon, med.	⅛
Apricots, dried	4 halves	Mango	½ small
Banana	½ small	*Orange	1 small
Blackberries	1 cup	*Orange juice	½ cup
Raspberries	1 cup	Papaya	⅓ medium
*Strawberries	1 cup	Peach	1 medium
Blueberries	⅔ cup	Pear	1 small
*Cantaloupe (6" dia.)	¼	Pineapple	½ cup
Cherries	10 large	Pineapple juice	⅓ cup
Dates	2	Plums	2 medium
Figs, fresh	2 large	Prunes, dried	2 medium
Figs, dried	1 small	Raisins	2 tablesp.
*Grapefruit	½ small	*Tangerine	1 large
*Grapefruit juice	½ cup	Watermelon	1 cup

* Contains considerable amount of vitamin C (ascorbic acid).

Meat Exchanges List 4

One exchange contains: Protein 7 grams, fat 5 grams: 75 calories.

	Amount to Use
Meat and poultry (medium fat)	1 ounce
(Beef, lamb, pork, liver, chicken, etc.)	
Cold cuts (4½" × ⅛")	1 slice
Salami, minced ham, bologna, liver-wurst, luncheon loaf	
Frankfurters (8–9 per lb.)	1
Egg	1
Fish: Haddock, etc.	1 ounce
Salmon, tuna, crab, lobster	¼ cup
Shrimp, clams, oysters, etc.	5 small
Sardines	3 medium
Cheese, Cheddar type	1 ounce
Cottage	¼ cup
Peanut butter	2 tablespoons

NOTE: Three meat exchanges are usually prescribed for the main meal of the day. This would be equal to ¼ lb. of meat or fish (raw weight) or three servings of any of the items listed above.

Bread Exchanges List 5

One exchange contains: carbohydrate 15 grams, protein 2 grams: 70 calories.

	Amount to Use
Bread...............................	1 slice
Biscuit, roll (2″ dia.)....................	1
Muffin (2″ dia.)	1
Cornbread (1½″ cube)...................	1
Cereals, cooked.........................	½ cup
Dry, flake and puff types................	¾ cup
Rice, grits, cooked......................	½ cup
Spaghetti, noodles, cooked................	½ cup
Macaroni, etc., cooked...................	½ cup
Crackers, graham (2½″ sq.)................	2
Oyster (½ cup)........................	20
Saltines (2″ sq.).......................	5
Soda (2½″ sq.).....·...................	3
Round, thin..........................	6
Flour................................	2½ tablespoons
Vegetables	
Beans and peas, dried, cooked (lima, navy, split pea, cowpeas, etc.).........	½ cup
Baked beans, no pork..................	¼ cup
Corn................................	⅓ cup
Popcorn.............................	1 cup
Parsnips.............................	⅔ cup
Potatoes, white.......................	1 small
Potatoes, white, mashed.................	½ cup
Potatoes, sweet or yams.................	¼ cup
Sponge cake, plain (1½″ cube).............	1
Ice cream............................	½ cup

(Omit two fat exchanges)

Fat Exchanges List 6

One exchange contains: Fat 5 grams: 45 calories.

	Amount to Use		Amount to Use
Butter or margarine..	1 teaspoon	French dressing.....	1 tablespoon
Bacon, crisp........	1 slice	Mayonnaise........	1 teaspoon
Cream, light........	2 tablespoons	Oil or cooking fat...	1 teaspoon
Cream, heavy.......	1 tablespoon	Nuts..............	6 small
Cream cheese.......	1 tablespoon	Olives.............	5 small
Avocado (4″ diameter) ⅛			

Diet No. 2

Carbohydrate 150 Gm., protein 70 Gm., fat 70 Gm.
Calories 1500

TOTAL DAY'S FOOD

List 1...............Milk, 1 pint
List 2A.............Vegetables, as desired
List 2B.............Vegetables, 1 serving
List 3...............Fruits, 3 servings
List 4...............Meat Exchanges, 6 servings
List 5...............Bread Exchanges, 6 servings
List 6...............Fat Exchanges, 4 servings

Select each day one green or yellow vegetable. One fruit or vegetable should be a good source of vitamin C.

This food may be divided into meals as follows:

SAMPLE MENU

Breakfast:
  Orange Juice—½ cup
  Egg—1
  Toast—1 slice   Butter—1 teaspoon
  Coffee—2 tablespoons light cream

Lunch or Supper:
  Ham and Cheese Sandwich
        (Cheese—1 ounce, Ham—1 ounce,
        Bread—2 slices, Butter—1 teaspoon)
  Lettuce and Tomato Salad
  Apple—1 small
  Milk—1 cup (8 ounces)
  Coffee or Tea

Dinner:
  Hamburg Patties—3 ounces
  Mashed Potato—½ cup
  Carrots—½ cup   Spinach
  Bread—1 slice   Butter—1 teaspoon
  Banana—½ small
  Coffee or Tea

Bedtime:
  Milk—1 cup (8 ounces)
  Graham Crackers—2

SAMPLE MEAL PLAN

Breakfast

Fruit, 1 serving....................List 3
Egg, or other meat exchange........List 4
Bread, 1 exchange..................List 5
Butter, 1 level teaspoon or other fat
    exchange.......................List 6
Tea or coffee......................As desired

Lunch or Supper

Meat, 2 exchanges..................List 4
Bread, 2 exchanges.................List 5
Vegetables, as desired.............List 2A
Fruit, 1 serving...................List 3
Milk, 1 cup........................List 1*
Butter, 1 level teaspoon or other fat
    exchange.......................List 6
Tea or coffee......................As desired

Dinner or main meal

Meat, 3 exchanges..................List 4
Bread, 2 exchanges.................List 5
Vegetables, as desired.............List 2A
Vegetables, 1 serving, $\frac{1}{2}$ cup........List 2B
Fruit, 1 serving...................List 3
Butter, 1 level teaspoon or other fat
    exchange.......................List 6
Tea or coffee......................As desired

Bedtime

Milk, 1 cup........................List 1*
Bread, 1 exchange..................List 5
Butter, 1 level teaspoon or other fat
    exchange.......................List 6

* Part of milk may be used in morning for coffee or for cereal when selected as a bread exchange.

Table 26.—Composition of Foods, 100 Grams, Edible Portion*

(Extracted, by permission, from Watt and Merrill: Composition of Foods, United States Department of Agriculture Handbook No. 8, 1950)

Food and description	Protein, Gm.	Fat, Gm.	Carbohydrate Total, Gm.
Almonds, dried, unblanched	18.6	54.1	19.6
Apples, Raw	.3	.4	14.9
Applesauce, canned: Unsweetened	.2	.2	10.9
Apricots: Raw	1.0	.1	12.9
Canned: Water pack, solids and liquid	.5	.1	8.1
Frozen	.7	.1	21.0
Asparagus, cooked	2.4	.2	3.6
Avocados, raw[1]	1.7	26.4	5.1
Bacon, medium fat:			
Broiled or fried, drained	25.	55.	.1
Bananas, raw	1.2	.2	23.
Beans, common or kidney, mature dry seeds:			
Red kidney, Raw, dry	23.1	1.7	59.4
Canned (or cooked) solids and liquid	5.7	.4	16.4
Other (including navy, pea, white marrow, other):			
Canned, baked: Pork and molasses	5.8	3.0	19.2
Beans, lima, Immature seeds: cooked	5.0	.4	18.3
Beans, snap:			
Green: Cooked (small amount of water, short time)	1.4	.2	4.7
Wax or yellow: Canned:			
Solids and liquid	1.0	.1	4.2
Drained solids	1.4	.2	4.7

Food and description	Protein, Gm.	Fat, Gm.	Carbohydrate Total, Gm.
Beef cuts, medium fat:			
Chuck: Cooked	26.	22.	0.
Hamburger: Cooked	22.	30.	0.
Porterhouse: Cooked	23.	27.	0.
Rib roast: Cooked	24.	24.	0.
Round: Cooked	27.	13.	0.
Sirloin: Cooked	23.	22.	0.
Beef, canned: Corned beef hash	13.7	6.1	7.2
Beef, corned, boneless:			
Canned: Medium fat	25.3	12.	0.
Beef, dried or chipped	34.3	6.3	0.
Beer (average, 4 per cent alcohol)[2]	.6		4.4
Beets, common red: Cooked	1.0	.1	9.8
Beet greens, common: Cooked	2.0	.3	5.6
Beverages, carbonated:			
Ginger ale	—	—	9.
Other, including kola type	—	—	12.
*Biscuits, baking powder, made with:			
Enriched flour	8.2	10.6	52.2
Blackberries:			
Raw	1.2	1.0	12.5
Canned, solids and liquids:			
Water pack	.9	.7	9.4
Blueberries:			
Raw	.6	.6	15.1

(287)

TABLE 26.—(Continued)

Food and description	Protein, Gm.	Fat, Gm.	Carbohydrate Total, Gm.
Bluefish: Cooked, baked	27.4	4.2	0.
Brains, all kinds, raw	10.4	8.6	.8
Bran (breakfast cereal, almost wholly bran)	12.0	3.4	74.2
Bran flakes (40 per cent bran)	10.8	1.9	78.8
Brazil nuts	14.4	65.9	11.0
*Breads:			
Boston brown bread made with de-germed corn meal: Unenriched	4.8	2.1	46.0
Cracked-wheat bread, made with:			
Enriched flour	8.5	2.2	51.4
Toasted	9.8	2.5	59.5
French or vienna breads: Enriched	8.1	2.7	52.0
Raisin bread: Unenriched	7.1	3.1	57.8
Toasted	7.9	3.5	64.6
Rye bread, American (1/3 rye, 2/3 clear flour)	9.1	1.2	52.4
White bread, Unenriched:			
4 per cent nonfat milk solids[3]	8.5	3.2	51.8
Toasted	9.7	3.7	59.0
White bread, enriched:			
4 per cent nonfat milk solids[3]	8.5	3.2	51.8
Toasted	9.7	3.7	59.0
Whole-wheat bread	9.3	2.6	49.0
Broccoli, flower stalks: Cooked	3.3	.2	5.5
Brussels sprouts: Cooked	4.4	.5	8.9
Buckwheat flour: Dark	11.7	2.5	72.0

Food and description	Protein, Gm.	Fat, Gm.	Carbohydrate Total, Gm.
Buckwheat flour: Light	6.4	1.2	79.5
Butter	.6	81.	.4
Buttermilk, cultured (made from skim milk)			
Cabbage: Raw	3.5	.1	5.1
Cooked (small amount of water, short time)	1.4	.2	5.3
Cabbage, celery or chinese: Raw	1.4	.2	5.3
	1.2	.3	2.4
*Cakes:			
Fruit, dark	5.2	13.8	55.9
Plain cake and cupcakes	6.4	8.2	57.0
Pound	7.1	23.5	49.3
Sponge	7.9	5.0	54.4
Candy:			
*Butterscotch	0.	8.9	85.6
*Caramels	2.9	11.6	77.5
Chocolate, sweetened, milk	(6.)	33.5	55.7
Chocolate, sweetened, milk, with almonds	(8.)	38.6	50.0
Chocolate creams	4.	14.	72.
*Fudge, plain	1.7	11.3	81.3
Hard	0.	0.	99.
Marshmallows	3.	0.	81.
*Peanut brittle	8.3	15.5	72.8
Cantaloups, raw	.6	.2	4.6
Carrots: Raw	1.2	.3	9.3
Cooked	.6	.5	6.4

Food and description	Protein, Gm.	Fat, Gm.	Carbohydrate Total, Gm.
Cashew nuts, roasted or cooked	18.5	48.2	27.0
Cauliflower: Raw	2.4	.2	4.9
Cooked	2.4	.2	4.9
Celery, bleached: Raw	1.3	.2	3.7
Cooked	1.3	.2	3.7
Chard, leaves and stalks: Cooked	1.4	.2	4.4
Cheese:			
Blue mold, domestic type	21.5	30.5	2.0
Camembert	17.5	24.7	1.8
Cheddar	25.0	32.2	2.1
Cheddar, processed	23.2	29.9	2.0
Cottage, from skim milk	19.5	.5	2.0
Cream cheese	9.0	37.0	2.0
Swiss	27.5	28.0	1.7
Cherries, sour, sweet, and hybrid, raw	1.1	.5	14.8
Chicken: Raw:			
Broilers, total edible	20.2	7.2	0.
Roasters, total edible	20.2	12.6	0.
Hens, total edible	18.0	25.0	0.
Chili sauce	2.8	0.4	23.7
Chocolate: Bitter or unsweetened	(5.5)	52.9	29.2[4]
Sweetened: Plain	(2.)	29.8	62.7
Milk. See Candy.			
Chocolate sirup	(1.2)	1.1	56.6
Clams, long and round: Raw, meat only	12.8	1.4	3.4
Cocoa, breakfast, plain, dry powder	(8.)	23.8	48.9
*Cocoa beverage, made with all milk	3.8	4.6	10.9

Food and description	Protein, Gm.	Fat, Gm.	Carbohydrate Total, Gm.
Coconut: Fresh, meat	3.4	34.7	14.0
Dried, shredded (sweetened)	3.6	39.1	53.2
Cod: Raw	16.5	.4	0.
Dried	81.8	2.8	0.
*Coleslaw	1.3	6.1	7.7
Collards: Cooked (boiled in small or moderate amount of water until tender)	3.9	.6	7.2
Cookies, plain and assorted	6.0	12.7	75.0
Corn, sweet, white or yellow: Cooked	2.7	.7	20.2
*Corn bread or muffins, made with:			
Enriched, degermed corn meal	6.7	4.7	36.6
Corn flakes	8.1	.3	85.0
Corn flour	7.8	2.6	76.8
Corn grits, degermed: Unenriched: Dry	8.7	.8	78.1
Corn meal, white or yellow:			
Degermed, unenriched: Dry	7.9	1.2	78.4
Crabs, Atlantic and Pacific, hardshell:			
Raw	16.1	1.6	.6
Crackers: Graham	8.0	10.0	74.3
Saltines	9.2	11.8	71.1
Soda, plain	9.6	9.6	72.7
Cranberries: Raw	.4	.7	11.3
Cranberry sauce, sweetened, canned or cooked	.1	.3	51.4
Cream: Light, table or coffee	2.9	20.0	4.0
Heavy or whipping	2.3	35.0	3.2
Cress, garden: Raw	4.2	1.4	5.3

19

TABLE 26.—(Continued)

Food and description	Protein, Gm.	Fat, Gm.	Carbohydrate Total, Gm.
Cucumbers, raw	.7	.1	2.7
Currants, red, raw	1.2	.2	13.6
*Custard, baked	5.3	5.4	11.2
Dandelion greens: Cooked	2.7	.7	8.8
Dates, "fresh" and dried	2.2	.6	75.4
Doughnuts, cake type	6.6	21.0	52.7
Eggplant, raw	1.1	.2	5.5
Eggs, hen, fresh, stored, or frozen: Raw:			
Whole	12.8	11.5	.7
White	10.8	0.	.8
Yolk	16.3	31.9	.7
Cooked:			
*Scrambled	11.0	12.8	2.2
Poached	12.7	11.4	.6
Endive, raw	1.6	.2	4.0
Farina, unenriched, raw	10.9	.8	77.4
Figs: Raw	1.4	.4	19.6
Dried	4.0	1.2	68.4
Fig bars	4.2	4.8	75.8
Flounder, summer and winter, raw	14.9	.5	0.
Fruit cocktail, canned, solids and liquid	.4	.2	18.6
Gelatin, dry: Plain	85.6	.1	0.
Dessert powder	9.4	0.	88.7
*Gelatin dessert, ready-to-serve: Plain	1.6	0.	15.2
With fruit added	1.4	.1	17.5
*Gingerbread	3.9	12.0	51.6
Grapefruit: Raw	.5	.2	10.1

Food and description	Protein, Gm.	Fat, Gm.	Carbohydrate Total, Gm.
Grapefruit: Canned in sirup, solid, liquid	.6	.2	19.1
Grapefruit juice: Fresh	.5	.1	9.2
Canned: Unsweetened	.5	.1	9.8
Sweetened	.5	.1	13.7
Grapefruit juice concentrate, frozen	1.9	.4	38.1
Grapefruit-orange juice blend: Canned:			
Unsweetened	.6	.1	10.4
Sweetened	.5	.1	13.9
Frozen concentrate	2.2	.4	37.9
Grapes, raw:			
American type (slip skin) as Concord, Delaware, Niagara, and Scuppernong	1.4	1.4	14.9
European type (adherent skin) as Malaga, Muscat, Sultanina (Thompson Seedless), and Flame Tokay	.8	.4	16.7
Grape juice, bottled, commercial	.4	.0	18.2
Guavas, common, raw	1.0	.6	17.1
Haddock: Raw	18.2	.1	0.
Cooked, fried	18.7	5.5	7.0
Halibut: Raw	18.6	5.2	0.
Cooked, broiled	26.2	7.8	0.
Herring, Atlantic, raw	18.3	12.5	0.
Herring, lake, raw	18.5	6.8	0.
Herring, Pacific, raw	16.6	2.6	0.
Herring, smoked, kippered	22.2	12.9	0.
Honey, strained or extracted	.3	0.	79.5
Honeydew melon, raw	.5	0.	8.5

Food and description	Protein, Gm.	Fat, Gm.	Carbohydrate Total, Gm.
Ice cream, plain	4.0	12.5	20.6
Jams, marmalades, preserves	.5	.3	70.8
Jellies	.2	0.	65.0
Kale, cooked	3.9	.6	7.2
Kidneys, raw: Beef	15.0	8.1	.9
Kohlrabi, cooked	2.1	.1	6.7
Lamb: Retail items,[5] medium fat:			
Rib chop, cooked	24.	35.	0.
Shoulder roast (wholesale 3-rib), cooked	21.	28.	0.
Leg roast (wholesale leg), cooked	24.	19.	0.
Lard	0.	100.	0.
Lemons	.9	.6	8.7
Lemon juice: Fresh	.4	.2	7.7
Canned: Unsweetened	.4	.2	7.7
Concentrate	2.0	1.0	37.5
Lentils, dry: Whole (entire seeds)	25.0	1.0	59.5
Lettuce, raw: Headed	1.2	.2	2.9
All other	1.2	.2	2.9
Limes	.8	.1	12.3
Lime juice, fresh	.4	.0	8.3
Liver: Beef: Cooked, fried	23.6	7.7	9.7
Lobster: Raw	16.2	1.9	.5
Canned	18.4	1.3	.4
Loganberries, raw	1.0	.6	15.0
Macaroni, Unenriched: Dry	12.8	1.4	76.5
*Cooked	5.1	.6	30.2

Food and description	Protein, Gm.	Fat, Gm.	Carbohydrate Total, Gm.
*Macaroni and cheese, baked	8.1	11.0	19.7
Mackerel: Raw, common Atlantic	18.7	12.	0.
Mangos, raw	.7	.2	17.2
Margarine	.6	81.	.4
Milk, cow:			
Fluid (pasteurized and raw):			
Whole	3.5	3.9	4.9
Nonfat (skim)	3.5	.1	5.1
Canned:			
Evaporated (unsweetened)	7.0	7.9	9.9
Condensed (sweetened)	8.1	8.4	54.8
Dried:			
Whole	25.8	26.7	38.0
Nonfat solids (skim)	35.6	1.0	52.0
Malted:[6]			
Dry powder	14.6	8.5	70.7
*Beverage	4.6	4.4	11.8
*Chocolate flavored	3.2	2.2	10.6
Milk, goat, fluid	3.3	4.0	4.6
Molasses, cane:			
Second extraction or medium	—	—	60.7
*Muffins, made with: Enriched flour	8.0	8.4	42.1
Mung bean sprouts, raw	2.9	.2	4.1
Mushrooms: Canned, solids and liquid	1.4	.2	3.7
Mustard greens, cooked	2.3	.3	4.0
Noodles (containing egg): Unenriched:			
Dry	12.6	3.4	73.2

TABLE 26.—(Continued)

Food and description	Pro-tein, Gm.	Fat, Gm.	Carbo-hydrate Total, Gm.
Noodles: *Cooked	2.2	.6	12.8
Oatmeal or rolled oats: Dry	14.2	7.4	68.2
*Cooked	2.3	1.2	11.0
Oils, salad or cooking	0.	100.	0.
Okra, cooked	1.8	.1	7.4
Olives, pickled: Green	1.5	13.5	4.0
Ripe: Mission	1.8	21.0	2.6
Other varieties (as ascalano, man-zanilla, and sevilano)	1.2	13.5	3.1
Onions, mature: Raw	1.4	0.2	10.3
Cooked	1.0	.2	8.7
Onions, young, green	1.0	.2	10.6
Oranges	.9	.2	11.2
Orange juice: Fresh	.8	.2	11.0
Canned: Unsweetened	.8	.2	11.1
Sweetened	.6	.2	13.9
Orange juice concentrate: Canned	4.2	.7	58.0
Frozen	2.7	.7	37.1
Oysters, meat only, raw	9.8	2.1	5.6
*Oyster stew: 1 part oysters to 3 parts milk by volume	5.3	5.4	5.3
*Pancakes (griddlecakes), baked:			
Wheat (home recipe):			
With unenriched flour	6.8	9.2	26.6
Buckwheat, with buckwheat pancake mix	6.1	8.4	20.9
Papayas, raw	.6	.1	10.0

Food and description	Pro-tein, Gm.	Fat, Gm.	Carbo-hydrate Total, Gm.
Parsley, common, raw	3.7	1.0	9.0
Parsnips, cooked	1.0	.5	13.9
Peaches: Raw	.5	.1	12.0
Canned, solids and liquid: Water pack	.5	.1	6.8
Frozen	.4	.1	20.2
Dried, sulfured: Uncooked	3.0	.6	69.4
Peanuts, Virginia type, roasted, shelled	26.9	44.2	23.6
Peanut butter	26.1	47.8	21.0
Pears: Raw	.7	.4	15.8
Canned, solids and liquid: Water pack	.3	.1	8.2
Peas, green, immature: Cooked	4.9	.4	12.1
Canned, solids and liquid	3.4	.4	12.9
Frozen	5.7	.3	12.9
Peas, mature dry seeds:			
Split, without seed coat	24.5	1.0	61.7
Pecans	9.4	73.0	13.0
Peppers, green, raw	1.2	.2	5.7
Cooked, parboiled then baked	1.3	.2	6.0
Persimmons, Japanese or Kaki, raw	.8	.4	20.0
Pickles: Dill, cucumber	.7	.2	2.1
Fresh, cucumber (as bread and butter pickles)	.9	.2	17.0
Sour, cucumber or mixed	.5	.2	2.2
Sweet, cucumber or mixed	.8	.4	26.4
Pies:			
*Apple	2.1	9.5	39.5
*Blueberry	2.1	6.9	37.5

Food and description	Pro-tein, Gm.	Fat, Gm.	Carbo-hydrate Total, Gm.
Pies: *Cherry	2.4	9.8	40.4
Custard	5.2	8.7	26.3
Lemon meringue	3.6	10.1	37.4
Mince8	2.5	6.9	45.6
*Pumpkin	4.2	9.6	25.8
Pineapple: Raw	.4	.2	13.7
Canned, sirup pack, solids and liquid	.4	.1	21.1
Pineapple juice, canned	.3	.1	13.0
Plantain or baking banana, raw	1.1	.4	31.2
Plums (all, excluding prunes), raw	.7	.2	12.9
Plums (Italian prunes), canned: Sirup pack, solids and liquid (except pits)	.4	.1	20.4
Popcorn, popped	12.7	5.0	76.7
Pork, fresh:			
Retail items,9 medium fat:			
Ham, cooked	24.	33.	0.
Loin or chops, cooked	23.	26.	0.
Pork, cured:			
Ham, smoked,10 medium fat: Cooked	23.	33.	(.4)
Luncheon meat, canned, spiced	14.9	24.3	1.5
Potatoes: Cooked:			
Baked	2.4	.1	22.5
Boiled, peeled before cooking	2.0	.1	19.1
*French-fried	5.4	19.1	52.0
*Hash-browned after holding overnight	3.3	11.7	31.9
*Mashed, milk added	2.2	.7	17.0

Food and description	Pro-tein, Gm.	Fat, Gm.	Carbo-hydrate Total, Gm.
Potato chips	6.7	37.1	49.1
Pretzels	8.8	3.2	74.5
Prunes, dried, unsulfured: Uncooked	2.3	.6	71.0
*Cooked, no sugar added	1.1	.3	33.0
Prune juice, canned	.4	0.	19.3
Pumpkin, canned	1.0	.3	7.9
Radishes, raw	1.2	.2	7.3
Raisins, unsulfured: Dried	2.3	.1	71.2
Raspberries: Black, raw	1.5	.5	15.7
Red: Raw	1.2	1.6	13.8
Frozen	.8	.4	24.7
Rhubarb, stems only: Raw	.5	.3	3.8
Rice: Brown, raw	7.5	.1	77.7
White or milled: Raw	7.6	1.7	79.4
*Cooked	2.5	.3	26.2
Rice products: Puffed	5.9	.6	87.7
*Rolls: Plain, enriched (pan rolls)	9.0	5.5	55.1
Rutabagas, cooked	.8	.1	7.5
Rye flour, dark	16.3	2.6	68.1
Rye wafers or "Swedish health bread"	12.4	1.2	75.3
Salad dressings:			
Commercial, plain (mayonnaise type)11	1.1	36.8	13.9
French	.6	35.5	20.3
Mayonnaise11	1.5	78.5	3.0
Salmon: Raw, Pacific (Chinook or King)	17.4	16.5	0.
Canned, solids and liquid (incl. bones): average	20.6	8.5	0.

Table 26.—(Continued)

Food and description	Protein, Gm.	Fat, Gm.	Carbohydrate Total, Gm.
Sardines: Atlantic type, canned in oil:			
Drained solids	25.7	11.0	1.2
Sauerkraut, canned: Drained solids	1.4	.3	4.4
Sausage:			
Bologna	14.8	15.9	3.6
Frankfurter, cooked	14.	20.	2.
Liver, liverwurst	16.7	20.6	1.5
Pork, links or bulk, raw	10.8	44.8	0.
Scallops, raw (edible muscle)	14.8	.1	3.4
Shad or American shad, raw	18.7	9.8	0.
*Sherbet	1.5	.0	30.0
Shrimp, canned:			
Dry pack or drained solids of wet pack	26.8	1.4	—
Sirup, table blends (chiefly corn sirup)	(0)	(0)	(74.)
Soups, canned:[12]			
Bean, ready-to-serve	3.4	2.0	11.8
Beef, ready-to-serve	2.4	1.4	4.4
Bouillon, broth, and consommé:			
Ready-to-serve	(1.)	—	(0)
Chicken, ready-to-serve	1.4	1.0	3.8
Clam chowder, ready-to-serve	1.8	.9	4.9
Cream soup (asparagus, celery, or mushroom), ready-to-serve	2.8	4.6	7.2
Pea, ready-to-serve	2.6	.8	10.2
Tomato, ready-to-serve	.9	.9	7.3
Vegetable, ready-to-serve	1.7	.7	5.8
Soybeans, whole, mature, dried	34.9	18.1	34.8[13]

Food and description	Protein, Gm.	Fat, Gm.	Carbohydrate Total, Gm.
Soybean flour, flakes, grits: Medium fat	42.5	6.5	37.2[13]
Spaghetti, unenriched: Dry	12.8	1.4	76.5
*Cooked	5.1	.6	30.2
Spinach: Raw	2.3	.3	3.2
Cooked	3.1	.6	3.6
Squash, summer: Cooked, diced	1.6	.1	3.9
Squash, winter: Cooked, boiled, mashed	1.5	.3	8.8
Starch, pure (including arrowroot, corn, etc.)			87.
Strawberries: Raw	.5	.2	8.3
Frozen	.8	.5	26.6
Sugars: Granulated, cane or beet	.6	.4	99.5
Powdered	(0.)	(0.)	99.5
Brown	(0.)	(0.)	95.5
Maple	—	—	(90.)
Sweet potatoes:[14] Cooked:			
Baked	2.2	.9	34.4
Boiled	1.8	.7	27.9
Swordfish, Cooked, broiled	27.4	6.8	0.
Tangerines (including other Mandarin type oranges)	.8	.3	10.9
Tapioca, dry	.6	.2	86.4
Tomatoes: Raw	1.0	.3	4.0
Canned or cooked	1.0	.2	3.9
Tomato juice, canned	1.0	.2	4.3
Tomato catsup	2.0	.4	24.5
Tomato purée, canned	1.8	.5	7.2

Food and description	Protein, Gm.	Fat, Gm.	Carbohydrate Total, Gm.
Tongue, beef, medium fat, raw	16.4	15.	.4
Tuna fish, canned: Drained solids	29.0	8.2	0.
Turkey, medium fat, raw	20.1	20.2	0.
Turnips, cooked	.8	.2	6.0
Turnip greens: Cooked: Boiled in small amount of water until tender	2.9	.4	5.4
Veal: Carcass or side excluding kidney fat, raw: Medium fat	19.1	12.	0.
Retail items,[15] medium fat: Cutlet, boned (wholesale round): Cooked	28.	11.	0.
Shoulder roast, boned (wholesale chuck): Cooked	28.	12.	0.
Vegetables, mixed, strained, canned (infant food)	1.6	.1	6.9
Vinegar	0.	—	(5.0)
*Waffles, baked: With unenriched flour	9.3	10.6	37.8
Walnuts, Persian or English	15.0	64.4	15.6
Watermelons	.5	.2	6.9

Food and description	Protein, Gm.	Fat, Gm.	Carbohydrate Total, Gm.
Wheat flours: Whole (from hard wheats)	13.3	2.0.	71.0
Patent: All-purpose or family flour: Unenriched	10.5	1.0	76.1
Enriched	10.5	1.0	76.1
Bread flour: Unenriched	11.8	1.1	74.7
Cake or pastry flour	7.5	.8	79.4
Wheat products: Flakes	10.8	1.6	80.2
Flakes (added iron, thiamine, and niacin)	10.8	1.6	80.2
Germ	25.2	10.0	49.5
Puffed	10.8	1.6	80.2
Puffed (added iron, thiamine, and niacin)	10.8	1.6	80.1
Shredded, plain	10.1	2.5	
Whey, fluid	.9	.3	5.1
Yeast: Compressed, baker's	(10.6)	.4	13.0
Dried, brewer's	(36.9)	1.6	37.4

* Asterisk indicates that values are calculated from a recipe; parentheses indicate imputed value.

1 Data on proximate constituents apply to Fuerte variety.

2 The value excluding energy derived from alcohol is 20 calories. If the energy from alcohol is considered available, the value is 48 calories.

3 When the amount of nonfat milk solids in commercial bread is unknown, use bread with 4 per cent nonfat milk solids, item 135 for unenriched bread and 139 for enriched.

TABLE 26.—(Continued)

⁴ Approximately one-third of this total amount of carbohydrate calculated by difference in starch and sugar. The remaining portions made up of materials thought to be utilized only poorly if at all by the body.

⁵ Values for raw items are from the medium fat wholesale cuts considered to be nearest approximations for indicated retail items.

⁶ Based on unfortified products.

⁷ Total sugars.

⁸ The proximate constituents, calcium, phosphorus, and vitamin A are calculated from a recipe.

⁹ Values for raw items are from medium fat wholesale cuts considered to be nearest approximations for indicated retail items.

¹⁰ Values for raw items are from the medium fat wholesale cuts considered to be nearest approximations for indicated retail items.

¹¹ Minerals and vitamins are calculated from a recipe.

¹² All the ready-to-serve soups are calculated from equal weights of the condensed soup and water except cream soup which was based on equal weights of the condensed soup and milk.

¹³ Approximately 40 per cent of this total amount of carbohydrate calculated by difference is sugar, starch, and dextrin. The remaining portion is made up of materials thought to be utilized only poorly, if at all, by the body.

¹⁴ If very pale varieties only were used, the vitamin A value would be very much lower.

¹⁵ Values for raw items are from the medium fat wholesale cuts considered to be nearest approximations for indicated retail items.

INDEX

(297)